HOUSE OFFI

Neurology

FIFTH EDITION

HOUSE OFFICER SERIES

Neurology

FIFTH EDITION

Howard L. Weiner, M.D.

Division of Neurology
Center for Neurologic Diseases
Brigham & Women's Hospital
Harvard Medical School
Boston, Massachusetts

Lawrence P. Levitt, M.D.

Division of Neurology
Lehigh Valley Hospital Center
Allentown, Pennsylvania

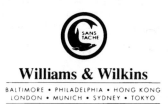

Williams & Wilkins

BALTIMORE • PHILADELPHIA • HONG KONG
LONDON • MUNICH • SYDNEY • TOKYO

A WAVERLY COMPANY

Editor: Timothy S. Satterfield
Managing Editor: Linda S. Napora
Copy Editor: Anne Schwartz
Cover Designer: Dan Pfisterer
Production Coordinator: Charles E. Zeller

Copyright © 1994
Williams & Wilkins
428 East Preston Street
Baltimore, Maryland 21202, USA

Accurate indications, adverse reactions, and dosage schedules for drugs are provided in this book, but it is possible that they may change. The reader is urged to review the package information data of the manufacturers of the medications mentioned.

Printed in the United States of America

First Edition 1973
Second Edition 1978
Third Edition 1983
Fourth Edition 1989

Library of Congress Cataloging-in-Publication Data

Weiner, Howard L.
    Neurology / Howard L. Weiner, Lawrence P. Levitt. — 5th ed. p. cm.
    (House officer series)

    Rev. ed. of: Neurology for the house officer. 4th ed. 1989.
    Includes bibliographical references and index.
    ISBN 0-683-08906-4
    1. Nervous system—Diseases—Handbooks, manuals, etc.
    2. Neurology—Handbooks, manuals, etc. I. Levitt, Lawrence P., 1940- .
    II. Weiner, Howard L. Neurology for the house officer. III. Title. IV.
    Series. [DNLM: 1. Nervous System Diseases. 2. Neurologic
    Manifestations.
WL 100 W424n 1993]
RC355.W44 1993
616.8—dc20
DNLM/DLC
for Library of Congress   93-12412
                                                                      CIP

                                                          96   97   98
                                                3   4   5   6   7   8   9   10

Dedication

To our wives, Mira and Eva

Foreword

Having spent my professional life in a teaching hospital with a steady stream of students, house officers, and residents, I have gradually become accustomed to the varying neurological backgrounds of these young physicians.

The neurologist and the internist exhibit significant differences in approach. The internist is usually trained to think physiologically in terms of the meaning and cause of specific symptoms. The neurologist, on the other hand, brings to the patient encounter not only his or her history and general physical examination, but a special "neurological examination." This special examination is designed more to answer the question "Where is the lesion?" than "What is wrong with the patient?"

In this country, most students and medical residents, general practitioners, and internists do not develop strong backgrounds in neurology. They therefore profit less from their neurological endeavors than they might. Nevertheless, they are still required to care for patients with nervous system disorders and are often significantly insecure about treatment.

In attempting to deal with this problem, Howard L. Weiner and Lawrence P. Levitt began compiling notes for their lectures to small groups of students. This soon became source material for future reference. The demand for this material grew geometrically, and their notes were widely used by students and residents. The need for a practical manual was appreciated, and the authors began a more systematic approach to problems with which they were recurrently faced on the wards of a large teaching hospital. As fast as they could put the sections out, students, medical interns, and residents kept requesting them, and soon large numbers were being duplicated. The material was recognized for its practical and common sense approach to frequently encountered problems.

After an intensive effort to gather constructive suggestions, find unmet needs, and weed out unimportant material, the authors wrote the first edition of this handbook 20 years ago.

Since its publication, *Neurology* (*House Officer Series*) has been enthusiastically received by physicians throughout the United States and has been published in several foreign language editions. It has become a standard guide for approaching neurological problems and its format has been the impetus for the creation of an entire series of house officer manuals in a variety of specialties.

I am certain that the fifth edition of this handbook will continue to meet the practical needs of physicians who care for patients with nervous system disorders.

H. Richard Tyler, M.D.

About the Authors

Howard L. Weiner, M.D., is Physician in Medicine (Neurology) at the Brigham and Women's Hospital and Robert L. Kroc Associate Professor of Neurologic Diseases at Harvard Medical School. He attended Dartmouth College and the University of Colorado Medical School; he then interned at Chaim Sheba Hospital, Tel Hashomer, Israel, and served as a medical resident at the Beth Israel Hospital, Boston. He received his neurology training at the Harvard teaching hospitals of the Longwood Area Neurology Program. Dr. Weiner is Director of the Multiple Sclerosis Clinical and Research Unit and Co-Director of the Center for Neurologic Diseases at the Brigham and Women's Hospital.

Lawrence P. Levitt, M.D., is Senior Consultant in Neurology at Lehigh Valley Hospital in Allentown, Pennsylvania. He is Clinical Professor of Neurology at Hahnemann University, and Clinical Associate Professor of Neurology at Temple University School of Medicine. A graduate of Queens College, he then attended Cornell Medical College as a Jonas Salk Scholar. Dr. Levitt interned and was a first-year medical resident at Bellevue Hospital and then spent 2 years in the Public Health Service at the Encephalitis Research Center in Tampa, Florida. He did his neurology training at the Harvard teaching hospitals of the Longwood Area Neurology Program.

With a Foreword by *H. Richard Tyler, M.D.*

H. Richard Tyler, M.D., is Professor of Neurology at Harvard Medical School and served as Head of the Section of Neurology at the Brigham and Women's Hospital for over 20 years. He serves as Consultant in Neurology for the Beth Israel Hospital, Children's Hospital, and the West Roxbury Veterans Administration Hospital. His responsibilities have included teaching students, interns and residents in the Harvard Medical

School for many years. He serves as Tutor in Neurology for the Harvard Medical School. Dr. Tyler is the author of numerous articles relating to the neurological aspects of disease.

This manual is designed to help physicians properly recognize and treat neurologic disease. It is not meant to be a complete survey but an attempt to outline succinctly the important clinical information about common neurologic problems. In the fifth edition we have added a new chapter on the neurology of other systemic diseases, updated references and treatment modalities, and included pertinent advances in neurologic diagnosis.

The approach is problem oriented: how to deal with a patient who is comatose, has a right hemiplegia, or is demented. We are most gratified by the widespread use of the previous editions of the manual and hope the fifth edition continues to fill the need for a readable, "carry in the pocket," practical reference to neurologic problems.

Howard L. Weiner, M.D.
Lawrence P. Levitt, M.D.

Acknowledgments

This manual was reviewed by students and house officers at the Harvard teaching hospitals of the Longwood Area Neurology Program and by members of the staff of Lehigh Valley Hospital. We are grateful to them for their encouragement, enthusiasm, and advice, and for identifying those neurologic problems and concepts most important to them. We would like to thank the following for their help and for reviewing parts of the manuscript: Doctors Barbara Dwaretsky, Frank Finch, Sally Kirkpatrick, Babu Krishnamurthy, Mark Osborne, and Marjorie Ross. We express particular appreciation to Marc Levitt who reviewed the manuscript and contributed the new chapter on the neurology of other systemic diseases.

Contents

The neurologic examination is designed to establish the localization of dysfunction in the nervous system. Many processes only affect specific areas in the nervous system...thus, anatomic localization becomes the foundation for both diagnosis and treatment.

Right-sided weakness may be secondary to a lesion affecting the pyramidal tract anywhere from cortex to spinal cord. Evaluation of associated signs and symptoms—e.g., aphasia with cortical lesions—is made to determine the level of the lesion.

Denial of illness and inattention of the left side are major features of nondominant hemisphere dysfunction. Tests of spatial organization and attention replace aphasia testing in evaluating patients with left hemiplegia.

Aphasia is the major feature of dominant hemisphere dysfunction. Recognition of asphasia establishes the level of nervous system involvement, and characterization may suggest the etiology.

Chapter 1

Localization

One of the major features of neurologic diagnosis is *localization of the lesion* in the nervous system. This approach is needed if one is consistently to arrive at reasonable diagnoses. Anatomic orientation is not merely an intellectual exercise; knowing where the lesion is will often indicate what it is, help guide in management, and be crucial in deciding on diagnostic procedures. Note the following examples.

PURE MOTOR HEMIPLEGIA

The nature of its anatomy usually defines the vascular lesion as a lacune and means that arteriography, anticoagulation, and surgery usually are not indicated. For more on pure motor hemiplegia, see Chapter 6.

MULTIPLE SCLEROSIS

Multiple lesions in the nervous system and a history of exacerbations and remissions are required for the diagnosis. When patients are misdiagnosed as having multiple sclerosis, there is often only one anatomic lesion.

HYSTERICAL SYMPTOMS

Hysteria is suspected when symptoms and/or signs do not fit anatomic rules.

FOOT-DROP

Foot-drop can be seen with peripheral nerve, nerve root, spinal cord, or hemisphere disease; one must decide where the dysfunction is before beginning investigation.

Knowledge of detailed neuroanatomy is usually not needed to decide whether the lesion is cortical, subcortical, in the brainstem, spinal cord, peripheral nerve, or muscle. When necessary, anatomic localization can be refined—first with the help of this manual, later with textbooks. If, after completing the history and physical examination, the physician begins the analysis by asking "Where is the lesion?," the major obstacle in making neurologic diagnoses will have been overcome.

Suggested Readings

Gilman S, Winans-Newman S. Manter & Gatz's essentials of clinical neuroanatomy and neurophysiology. 7th ed. Philadelphia: FA Davis, 1987.

Haymaker W. Bing's local diagnosis in neurological disease. St. Louis: CV Mosby, 1969.

Chapter 2

Right Hemiplegia

When examining a patient with right hemiplegia (paralysis) or right hemiparesis (weakness), establish whether the lesion is cortical, subcortical, in the brainstem, or in the spinal cord (Fig. 2.1).

IS THE LESION CORTICAL?

1. Test the patient carefully for *aphasia*. Have the patient name objects (e.g., pen, tie, watch), repeat phrases ("no ifs, ands, or buts"), read (a magazine or newspaper) and check for comprehension. Check writing. Listen carefully to spontaneous speech for aphasic errors. Is the patient right-handed? Remember, in nearly all right-handed and most left-handed people, the left hemisphere is dominant for speech (see Chapter 4, Aphasia).

2. Check for *cortical sensory loss*. Test position sense, point localization, graphesthesia (write numbers on the palm), and double simultaneous stimulation and stereognosis (using a coin, comb, or pen).

3. Are the *face and arm more involved than the leg* (suggesting middle cerebral artery territory), or is the leg more involved (anterior cerebral)?

4. Is there *eye deviation?* Eyes deviate toward the hemisphere involved and away from the hemiparesis in cortical lesions (See Fig. 31.2).

5. Check carefully for a *field defect*. Have the patient identify fingers presented simultaneously in peripheral fields. *Note:* Field defects and "cortical-type" eye deviation may be found in subcortical lesions and must be interpreted in the con-

Is the lesion

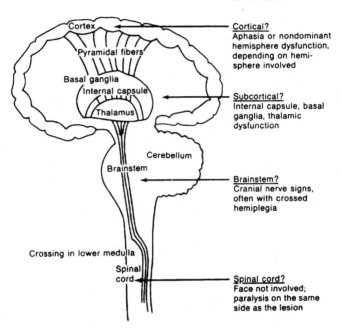

Cortical?
Aphasia or nondominant hemisphere dysfunction, depending on hemisphere involved

Subcortical?
Internal capsule, basal ganglia, thalamic dysfunction

Brainstem?
Cranial nerve signs, often with crossed hemiplegia

Spinal cord?
Face not involved; paralysis on the same side as the lesion

Figure 2.1. Establishing the level of the lesion in a patient with hemiplagia.

text of other findings. The presence of seizures, cortical sensory loss, or aphasia will often assist in accurate diagnosis.

6. Has the hemiparesis been associated with a seizure suggesting a cortical focus? Has the patient had seizures in the same distribution as the weakness?

IS THE LESION SUBCORTICAL?

Subcortical structures include the internal capsule, basal ganglia (globus pallidus and putamen), and thalamus.

1. Are *face, arm, and leg equally involved* (characteristic of lesions in the internal capsule)?
2. Are there dystonic postures (seen with lesions of the basal ganglia)?

3. Is there a *dense sensory loss* to pinprick and touch in face, arm, and leg (seen with thalamic lesions) associated with the hemiplegia? The latter is due to involvement of the adjacent internal capsule.

4. Is there *eye deviation* or a field defect as seen in cortical lesions?

IS THE LESION IN THE LEFT BRAINSTEM?

1. Look for *crossed hemiplegia,* a classic feature of brainstem lesions. Right hemiplegia from a left-sided brainstem lesion often produces left-sided brainstem signs (e.g., left-sided dysmetria or cranial nerve palsies) at the level of the lesion.

2. Check for *cerebellar signs:* finger-to-nose ataxia, difficulty with rapid alternating movements in the limbs, difficulty walking heel-to-toe (tandem gait). Remember, limb ataxia is almost always on the same side as the lesion, so a left brainstem lesion gives left limb ataxia. Do not misinterpret weakness for ataxia.

3. Note *nystagmus*. This is usually more marked when the patient gazes toward the side of the lesion.

4. Check for hearing loss in the left ear.

5. Check carefully for *sensory findings*. Characteristic findings are pain, temperature, and corneal loss on the left side of the face (involvement of descending tract of the fifth nerve) with pain and temperature loss on the right side of the body (spinothalamic tract).

6. Note *dysarthria* and *difficulty with swallowing*. Pseudobulbar palsy, often secondary to multiple bilateral vascular lesions above the brainstem, also causes dysarthria and dysphagia. The patient with pseudobulbar palsy, though, usually has a hyperactive rather than a decreased gag, brisk jaw jerk, emotional lability, and a history of previous strokes.

7. Check for abnormal *eye movements*. For example, patients with right hemiplegia secondary to left brainstem lesions may have trouble gazing to the left (see Fig. 31.2) or in getting the left eye to cross the midline when looking to the right (internuclear ophthalmoplegia) (see Fig. 31.7).

8. Tongue deviation is to the left with lesions of the left twelfth nerve or its nucleus, since the stronger right-sided hypoglossus muscle pushes the tongue to the left. Left-sided lesions above the nucleus (including the cortex) may cause tongue

deviation to the right, since supranuclear innervation is crossed. In ascertaining the extent of tongue deviation, use the tip of the nose as a point of reference for the midline.

IS THE LESION IN THE SPINAL CORD?

1. The *face* is usually not involved. Language function and cranial nerves are not involved.
2. *Paralysis* is on the same side as the lesion. *Pinprick and temperature* loss on the opposite side (Brown-Séquard's syndrome) may be seen (see Fig. 31.5).
3. A *sensory level* to pinprick, vibration, or a sweat level may be present.
4. *Bladder* and bowel disturbances are common.

Suggested Reading

Gilman S, Winans-Newman S. Manter & Gatz's essentials of clinical neuroanatomy and neurophysiology. 7th ed. Philadelphia: FA Davis, 1987.

Chapter 3

Left Hemiplegia

When examining a patient with a left hemiplegia, nondominant hemisphere function rather than aphasia testing is stressed. The remainder of cortical, subcortical, brainstem, and spinal cord testing is the same.

ARE THERE NONDOMINANT HEMISPHERE FINDINGS?

1. Check for *inattention.* Does the patient neglect the body's left side, the left side of the room, or the left side of a picture? Check for *extinction* by double simultaneous sensory or visual stimulation (touch both of the patient's hands at once and ask which was touched; have the patient identify fingers presented simultaneously in peripheral fields).
2. Check for *denial* or "*unconcern.*" Does the patient deny that anything is wrong, or, despite being aware of hemiplegia, show little concern? Sometimes, a patient will not recognize his or her own left hand when it is lifted into view.
3. Test for *constructional apraxia.* Have the patient attempt to copy a simple diagram (e.g., a cube) or designs made with tongue depressors. Have the patient draw a clock and fill in the numbers.
4. *Does the patient have difficulty dressing* (dressing apraxia)?
5. Check for *spatial disorientation* by leading the patient from the room: can he or she find the way back? Have the patient analyze a picture. Check topography by asking directions about local travel.
6. Is there *impersistence* at a task? Can the tongue be held out or an "ahhh" maintained?

7. Is there an acute confusional state, as has been reported in some patients with nondominant hemisphere strokes?
8. Check prosody by listening to the patient's voice (is it monotonous) and asking the patient to repeat a phrase with emotional content or interpret the emotional content of a sentence.

Suggested Readings

Critchley M. The parietal lobes. New York: Hafner, 1969.

Denny-Brown D, Chambers RA. The parietal lobe and behavior. Res Publ Assoc Res Nerv Ment Dis 1958;36:35.

Fisher CM. Left hemiplegia and motor impersistence. J Nerv Ment Dis 1956;123:201.

Mesulam M-M, Waxman S, Geschwind N, et al. Acute confusional states with right middle cerebral artery infarctions. J Neurol Neurosurg Psychiatry 1976;39:84.

Chapter 4

Aphasia

Aphasia is a disorder of language; the aphasic patient uses language incorrectly or comprehends it imperfectly. The dysarthric patient, on the other hand, articulates poorly, but grammar and word choice are correct. Aphasia must be recognized clinically because it localizes the lesion to the cortex (or immediately under the cortex) and to the left hemisphere. There are three exceptions:

1. Some (less than 50%) left-handed people use the right hemisphere for speech.
2. Anomic aphasias, where the inability to generate word names is the predominant feature, may result from metabolic disorders or space-occupying lesions with pressure effects.
3. Thalamic lesions, especially on the left, may produce aphasia.

Since different types of aphasia may imply different etiologies, the clinician must first be able to recognize that aphasia exists and then to characterize it.

ANATOMY OF APHASIA

Language "ability" is a function of the left hemisphere for almost all right-handed and for most left-handed individuals. The anatomic components of language are located primarily in the distribution of the middle cerebral artery surrounding the sylvian and rolandic fissures. Speech production involves four regions in this area, moving from posterior to anterior. Thus, speech connections exist between Wernicke's area or the posteri-

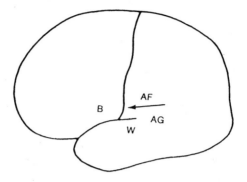

Figure 4.1.   The four regions of speech production. Moving from posterior to anterior, they are Wernicke's area (*W*) or the posterior part of the first temporal gyrus; the angular gyrus (*AG*); the arcuate fasciculus (*AF*); and Broca's area (*B*) or the posterior third frontal gyrus.

or part of the first temporal gyrus; the angular gyrus; the arcuate fasciculus; and Broca's area or the posterior third frontal gyrus.

Wernicke's area lies next to the primary auditory cortex and involves the "understanding" of auditory input as language and monitors speech output. It is connected with the *angular gyrus,* a center for integrating sensory and other association information.

The arcuate fasciculus is a white matter tract leading to *Broca's area,* which in turn is responsible for the motor part or " production" of language. Broca's area translates the information carried from other speech areas into phonation and actual speech.

FIVE TYPES OF A PHASIA

Broca's Aphasia

The lesion is in or near Broca's area.
1.   Speech is slow, *nonfluent,* produced with great effort, and poorly articulated. There is marked reduction in total speech, which may be "telegraphic" with the omission of small words or endings.
2.   *Comprehension* of written and verbal speech is good.
3.   *Repetition* of single words may be good, though it is done with

great effort; phrase repetition is poor, especially phrases containing small function words (e.g., "no ifs, ands, or buts").

4. The patient always *writes* in an aphasic manner, and writing is consistently affected even in a subtle aphasia.
5. *Object naming* is usually poor, although it may be better than spontaneous speech.
6. *Hemiparesis* (usually greater in the arm than the leg) is present, because the motor cortex is close to Broca's area.
7. The patient is *aware* of this deficit; he or she is frustrated and frequently depressed.
8. Interestingly, the patient may be able to hum a melody normally. However, if the patient is a musician and views music as a language, deficits in "producing" music will be experienced. Curses or other ejaculatory speech may be well articulated.
9. Buccolingual apraxia may be present.

Wernicke's Aphasia

The lesion is in or near Wernicke's area.

1. *Speech* is *fluent* with normal rhythm and articulation, but it conveys information poorly because of circumlocutions, use of empty words, and incorrect words (paraphasic errors).
2. The patient uses wrong words and sounds—i.e., making *paraphasic errors* and using neologisms ("treen" for train; "here is my clover" for here is my hand).
3. The patient is unable to *comprehend* written or verbal speech.
4. The content of *writing* is abnormal, as is speech, though the penmanship may be good.
5. *Repetition* is poor.
6. *Object naming* is poor.
7. *Hemiparesis* is mild or absent, since the lesion is far from the motor cortex. A hemianopsia or quadrantanopsia may be present.
8. Patients do not realize the nature of their deficit and usually are not depressed in the acute stage. They may exhibit elements of paranoia for this reason.
9. This type of aphasia is commonly the result of an embolic event to the superior temporal gyrus.

Conduction Aphasia

This is due to a temporal or parietal lesion involving the arcuate fasciculus and/or connecting fibers "disconnecting" Wernicke's and Broca's areas.

1. *Speech* is fluent but conveys information imperfectly. Paraphasic errors are common.
2. The patient can *comprehend* spoken or written phrases containing small grammatical words.
3. *Repetition* is the most severely affected, especially for phrases containing small grammatical words and nonsense syllables.
4. There is difficulty *naming objects.*
5. *Written language* is impaired, though penmanship is preserved.
6. *Hemiparesis,* if present, is usually mild.

Anomic Aphasia

1. This type of aphasia may be seen with small lesions in the angular gyrus, toxic or metabolic encephalopathies, or focal space-occupying lesions far from the speech area that exert pressure effects. It is the least localizing of the aphasias and should prompt a serious search for reversible, metabolic causes.
2. *Speech* is fluent but conveys information poorly because of paraphasic errors and circumlocutions (written language is impaired in the same way). Even though this aphasia is termed anomic aphasia (difficulty in naming objects), anomia is not unique to this type of aphasia.
3. The patient can *understand* both written and spoken speech.
4. There is no *hemiplegia.*
5. *Comprehension* and *repetition* are normal, although these may be difficult to assess in a patient who is confused.

Global Aphasia

This type of aphasia is seen with large lesions affecting both Wernicke's and Broca's areas. Marked hemiparesis occurs, plus inability to comprehend and to speak. Global aphasia is seen with large infarcts in the middle cerebral artery territory and is often due to occlusion of the left internal carotid artery or trunk of the middle cerebral artery.

Other Aphasic Syndromes

Broca's, Wernicke's, conduction, and global aphasias involve repetition difficulty because the lesion(s) involve the speech area in the perisylvian region. Less commonly, aphasias occur due to lesions located outside the perisylvian region, in "border zone" areas. Aphasic syndromes, such as isolation of the speech area, transcortical motor aphasia, and transcortical sensory aphasia, have been described (see Suggested Readings for detailed discussion). The clinical importance of transcortical aphasias is that they are typically related to prolonged hypotension or hypoxia, e.g., after cardiac arrest. These patients often repeat and read well but have diminished fluency (anterior border zone lesions) or comprehend poorly (posterior border zone lesions).

EXAMINATION OF THE APHASIC PATIENT

First establish whether the patient is in fact aphasic, then determine the nature of the aphasia. Remember, it may be difficult to determine whether an inattentive or confused patient is aphasic.

1. *Listen to speech output.* Is it fluent or nonfluent? If fluent, the lesion is posterior; if nonfluent, it usually is anterior.
2. Can the patient *read and write* with no errors? If so, aphasia is not present.
3. Is there *hemiparesis?* If so, the lesion is anterior, involving the motor area.
4. To delineate the various types of fluent aphasias, check whether the patient can repeat, comprehend, and name.
   - Wernicke's: cannot repeat or comprehend; names poorly
   - Conduction: cannot repeat but can comprehend; names poorly
   - Anomic: Can both repeat and comprehend but has trouble with naming.

THE IMPORTANCE OF DEFINING THE APHASIA

The definition of aphasia localizes the *level* of the nervous system lesion. If aphasia is present, the lesion is usually in the left cerebral cortex. Someone with difficulty using the right hand and a mild aphasia has hemisphere disease, not a brachial plexus lesion.

Aphasia implies dysfunction of middle cerebral artery territory and is often caused by disease of the internal carotid in the neck. Marked stenosis of the internal carotid may be surgically correctable, and if recognized and treated in time a mild or transient aphasia may be prevented from becoming global.

The sudden onset of fluent aphasia without hemiparesis often means an embolus to the posterior branch of the middle cerebral artery. Look for an embolic focus in the heart or in the carotid artery. If the heart is the source, anticoagulation should be considered; if the carotid is the suspected source, angiography is usually performed in search of a surgically remediable lesion. Remember the clinical rule: the sudden onset of aphasia without hemiparesis suggests embolus.

PROGNOSIS

The prognosis of aphasia in a given patient depends on the location and extent of the lesion. Patients with global aphasia have a poor prognosis and almost never recover completely. Patients with anomic, conduction, and transcortical aphasias have a good prognosis and complete recovery occurs frequently. Broca's and Wernicke's aphasia patients have an intermediate prognosis and show a wide range of outcomes. In general, patients with traumatic cases of aphasia do better than those in whom stroke is the cause. The bulk of evidence indicates that speech therapy improves the outcome in aphasia. New treatment techniques such as comprehension treatment programs and visual communication therapy are being employed to help the aphasic patient. Cooperation between the neurologist, speech pathologist and psychologist benefits the patient greatly. Note the following points.

1. *Apraxia* is a disturbance of purposeful movement that cannot be accounted for by elementary motor or sensory

impairments or by impaired comprehension or cooperation. For example, in dressing apraxia the patient is unable to dress despite adequate motor power. Apraxias occur commonly in association with aphasic syndromes and usually involve the "disconnection" of one brain area from another.

2. *Agnosias* are disorders of recognition that are not accounted for by elementary motor or perceptual disturbances. For example, visual agnosia is a disorder of recognition not accounted for by a primary disorder of vision.

3. Left posterior parietal disease (Gerstmann's syndrome) includes agraphia, left-right confusion, finger agnosia, and difficulty with calculations.

DISCONNECTION SYNDROMES

Disconnection syndromes occur when one part of the cortex is disconnected from the other. Examples include:

1. *Alexia without agraphia.* Patient can write but cannot read—lesion in the left occipital region and adjacent corpus callosum.

2. *Balint's syndrome.* Patient has visual inattention and cannot direct gaze to specific points in the visual field despite full extraocular movement (optic ataxia and visual apraxia)—bilateral parieto-occipital lesions.

3. *Pure word deafness.* Patient cannot interpret words or repeat what is said, but can hear and can interpret written language—deep left temporal lobe lesion.

4. *Ideomotor apraxia.* Patient uses left hand well for all functions except those suggested by verbal commands—lesion in left frontal cortex and adjacent corpus callosum.

Suggested Readings

Albert ML, Helm-Estabrooks N. Diagnosis and treatment of aphasia Part I, JAMA 1988;259:1043–1047(Part I); 1205–1210(Part II).

Benson DF, Geschwind N. Aphasia and related disturbances. In: Baker, Joynt, eds. Clinical neurology. New York: Harper & Row, 1988.

Damasio AR. Aphasia. N Engl J Med 1992;326:531–539.

Chapter 5

Stroke

Stroke is one of the most common neurologic problems confronting the internist. Some aspects of the treatment of stroke (embolus, thrombosis, hemorrhage) are controversial. This chapter presents a basic approach to the patient with stroke and outlines generally accepted modalities of treatment.

WHERE IS THE STROKE? WHAT IS THE ANATOMY?

Emboli tend to move peripherally, giving cortical deficits. *Intracranial hemorrhage* is usually deep and most commonly affects the putamen, thalamus, pons, or cerebellum. *Thrombosis* produces a wide variety of syndromes; diagnosis is based on history, anatomy of the deficit, and conclusion that embolus and hemorrhage are unlikely possibilities. *Lacunes* (see Chapter 6) may give characteristic anatomic deficits that identify the stroke. In *subarachnoid hemorrhage,* the neurologic deficit, if any, depends on where the bleeding occurs. See Table 5.1 for stroke types.

HOW DID THE STROKE DEVELOP?

Emboli usually give maximal deficit at onset and occur most often during waking hours. The deficit usually improves within 1 to 2 days, sometimes within hours. There usually is no warning. There may be headache and/or focal seizures.

Intracranial hemorrhage also occurs during waking hours, usually in a known hypertensive patient or in a patient with a bleeding tendency (e.g., a patient receiving anticoagulants). The full deficit is seldom present at onset but develops gradually over

Table 5.1.
Stroke Types

Infarct
    Thrombotic
    Embolic

Hemorrhage
    Intracerebral
    Subarachnoid

---

minutes to hours. There is no warning; headache, nausea, and vomiting are usually but not invariably present.

Thrombosis often occurs during sleep or is present upon arising in the morning. Symptoms and signs usually progress in a stepwise fashion; it may take hours or days for the full deficit to develop.

A warning is common in thrombotic strokes.

The patient often has a headache and frequently was warned of the attack with previous transient neurologic symptoms or a transient ischemic attack (TIA). A warning is common in thrombotic strokes and should always be diligently sought.

1. *TIAs in carotid distribution:* transient blindness in the eye on the same side as a narrowed internal carotid artery (amaurosis fugax). Patient may report a "shade coming down" over the eye, or "white steam."
   - Transient aphasia
   - Motor and sensory symptoms in a single extremity (upper or lower), or a clumsy "bear's paw" hand.
2. *TIAs in vertebrobasilar distribution:* slurred speech, dizziness, ataxia, syncope, dysphagia, numbness around lips or face, double vision.
   - Hemiparesis and hemi–sensory loss do not parallel each other in the individual limb as in carotid disease. There may be bilateral motor or sensory deficits from a single lesion.

Lacunar or small-vessel strokes occur abruptly or in a stuttering fashion over hours or days. There may be a warning; headache is absent; hypertension is usually present.

Subarachnoid hemorrhage occurs abruptly with severe headache as the cardinal feature, often coming on during physical exertion. It is often associated with stiff neck and photophobia.

WHAT ARE THE HISTORICAL CLUES AND PHYSICAL FINDINGS?

Is There Evidence for Occlusion or Narrowing of Internal or Common Carotid Artery?

1. Check for (*a*) decreased or absent pulsation of the carotid in the neck and (*b*) a bruit over the carotid.
2. Is there an increase in ipsilateral external carotid pulses in the face (superficial temporal, brow, angular), representing collateral circulation around an occluded internal carotid? Check for symmetry of these pulses between sides of the face.
3. A Horner's syndrome may be seen ipsilateral to a common carotid occlusion.
4. Patients with hypertension may have less hypertensive change in the fundus on the side of carotid narrowing.
5. In addition to the physical examination of the carotids, there are noninvasive tests currently available and widely used to help detect hemodynamically severe carotid lesions. Some of the more important include the following:
    a. Oculopneumoplethysmography (OPG) detects stenosis of hemodynamic consequence (75% cross-sectional area reduction or greater) from the level of the aortic arch to that of the carotid siphon. This is done by measuring the ophthalmic systolic pressure (the ophthalmic artery is the first branch of the internal carotid artery), and the brachial systolic pressure in a given patient and plotting this ratio against a standard regression line of normal values. With newer techniques, OPG is used less frequently.
    b. Duplex carotid ultrasound employs high-resolution B-mode scanning of the carotid to visualize plaque morphology directly and to measure various degrees of carotid stenosis and intraluminal area reduction. In addition, this technique uses Doppler spectral analysis to assess local characteristics of blood flow through various portions of the vessel and helps determine the degree of stenosis or occlusion.

c. Magnetic resonance angiography (MRA) is a computerized imaging modality that is sensitive to flowing blood. Surrounding tissues are not imaged, but arteries and/or veins are visualized much like routine arteriograms. The difference between the two is that in MRA there is no injection of a contrast agent; the study is purely noninvasive. Although images can be acquired of the veins and arteries of the head, the best results so far have been obtained with imaging the cervical carotid and vertebral arteries.

Recent studies have shown MRA to be extremely accurate in detecting atherosclerotic narrowing of the cervical carotid arteries. Also, unlike routine arteriography, most MRA scans can be acquired and displayed in three-dimensional view, allowing the physician to sit at a console and manipulate or evaluate the vessels in numerous projections.

d. Transcranial Doppler (TCD) is an ultrasound technology that measures blood flow in the major intracranial arteries. The technique records flow velocities in the carotid siphon through an orbital window, in the middle and posterior cerebral arteries through a temporal window and in the vertebrobasilar system through a foramen magnum window. TCD is of established value in (*a*) detecting severe stenosis (>65%) in the major basal intracranial arteries; (*b*) assessing the patterns of collateral circulation in patients with known regions of severe stenosis or occlusion; (*c*) evaluating and following patients with vasoconstriction of any cause, particularly after often subarachnoid hemorrhage; (*d*) detecting arteriovenous malformations (AVMs) and studying their major supply arteries and flow patterns; and (*e*) assessing intracranial velocity and flow changes in patients with suspected brain death.

Other uses of TCD such as monitoring during cerebral endarterectomy or coronary bypass are under investigation.

While cerebral arteriography remains the definitive method for visualizing the carotid circulation, the above noninvasive methods are playing an increasingly important role in the detection of cerebrovascular disease and the prevention of stroke.

6. Cholesterol emboli (shiny refractile bodies or Hollenhorst plaques) may be seen in the retinal arteries on the same side as a diseased carotid.

7. When dealing with stroke in young adults, pursue risk factors such as use of oral contraceptives, previously undetected hypertension, mitral valve prolapse, patent foramen ovale with paradoxical embolism, hypercoagulable states (antithrombin III deficiency, protein C deficiency, protein S deficiency, sickle cell anemia, familial plasminogen deficiency, lupus anticoagulant), and metabolic disorders (e.g., homocystinuria).

8. Cocaine abuse, regular alcohol consumption, and smoking are emerging as important causes of stroke, especially in the young adult. Stroke syndromes associated with cocaine include subarachnoid hemorrhage due to rupture of aneurysms and arteriovenous malformations, intracerebral hemorrhage, and cerebral infarction. Regular alcohol consumption is associated with hypertension, intracranial hemorrhage, cerebral infarction, and increased risk of death from stroke. Abuse of amphetamine has been associated with intracranial hemorrhage ("speed" hemorrhage).

Therefore, ask about drug and alcohol use in evaluating the stroke patient, especially in a young adult.

Large- or Small-Vessel Disease?

Warning symptoms tend to be stereotyped in small-vessel disease and occur over hours to days. In large-vessel disease the symptoms frequently vary depending on which territory of the vessel is involved during the warning; symptoms usually precede the stroke by days or weeks but may occur over a period of months. See Table 5.2 for cerebrovascular diseases that cause stroke.

Headache is common with large-vessel occlusion. Posterior circulation stroke often produces headache over the occiput, and anterior circulation stroke usually produces headache behind the eyes or over the forehead or temples. Headache rarely accompanies small-vessel occlusion.

Table 5.2.
Cerebrovascular Diseases That Cause Stroke

Atherosclerosis
Embolus
Lipohyalinosis (e.g., from hypertension)
Aneurysm (subarachnoid hemorrhage)
Arteriovenous malformation
Hypercoagulable state
Trauma (leading to dissection)
Vasculitis

Is There an Embolic Focus?

The *heart* is the most common source of emboli, though they may arise from a plaque in a diseased carotid artery or aorta. Cardiogenic emboli account for 15–20% of all ischemic strokes. *Cardiac factors* predisposing to emboli include mural thrombus associated with myocardial infarction (MI), especially anterior MIs or those associated with a hypodynamic left ventricle (emboli usually occur within 10 days but sometimes months after the MI and may be the presenting feature of an MI), mitral valve disease, and atrial fibrillation. Transesophageal echocardiography is proving to be a valuable aid in detecting cardiac mural thrombi as a source of cerebral emboli. Paroxysmal cardiac arrhythmias are an important cause of embolic stroke and may require a Holter monitor for detection. Other cardiac embolic risk factors include prosthetic or calcified valves, bacterial endocarditis, marantic endo-carditis, atrial myxoma, and cardiomyopathy.

NOTE: It is important to realize that there are exceptions to the above rules. Emboli can progress in a stepwise fashion, thrombosis can occur during the day, and hemorrhage may masquerade as thrombosis. Nevertheless, these rules are useful; when combined with other information about the patient, they help guide to the diagnosis. See Table 5.3 for characteristic features of stroke.

Table 5.3.
Characteristic Features of Stroke[a]

	Embolus	Intracerebral Hemorrhage	Large Vessel Thrombosis	Lacune	Subarachnoid Hemorrhage
Location	Peripheral (cortical)	Deep (basal ganglia, thalamus, cerebellum)	Variable (depends on vessel)	Pons, internal capsule	Vessels at junction of the circle of Willis
Onset	Sudden (maximum deficit at onset)	Sudden (deficit develops over minutes to hours)	Sudden, gradual, stepwise, or stuttering	Sudden, gradual, stepwise, or stuttering	Sudden, usually few or no focal signs
When	Awake	Awake and active	Asleep or inactive	Asleep or inactive	Asleep or inactive
Warning (TIA)	None	None	Usually	Variable, TIAs may occur	None
Headache	Sometimes	Usually	Sometimes	No	Always (stiff neck)
CT scan	Decreased density	Increased density	Decreased density	Decreased density	Usually normal
MRI T_1	Hypointense	b	Hypointense	Usually normal	Usually normal[a]
T_2	Hyperintense	b	Hyperintense	Hyperintense	Usually normal[a]
LP	Usually clear	Usually bloody	Clear	Clear	Invariably bloody

[a] These characteristics are generally accepted principles regarding stroke; however, remember they are not hard rules, and stroke can present atypically.

[b] The appearance of hemorrhage on MRI scan is variable and dependent on multiple factors, e.g., type of scan (T_1 versus T_2 weighted), location (intraparenchymal versus extradural versus subarachnoid) and time (acute, subacute, chronic). The interested reader should consult Bradley WG. MRI of hemorrhage and iron in the brain. In: Stark DD, Bradley WG. Magnetic Resonance Imaging. St. Louis: CV Mosby, 1988.

LABORATORY EXAMINATION

Laboratory investigation of the stroke patient should include:

- *Complete blood count:* blood dyscrasia polycythemia thrombo-cytopenia or thrombocytosis or infection as risk factors for stroke
- *Prothrombin time, partial thromboplastin time:* clue to the patient with antiphospholipid antibody (prolonged partial thromboplastin time)
- *Urinalysis:* hematuria in subacute bacterial endocarditis (SBE) with embolic stroke
- *Sedimentation rate:* elevation a clue to vasculitis, hyperviscosity or SBE as cause of stroke
- *Chemistry screen:* elevated blood glucose, cholesterol or triglyceride levels
- *Chest x-ray:* enlarged heart as embolic source of stroke or evidence of prolonged hypertension; may detect an unsuspected malignancy
- *Electrocardiogram:* may reveal arrhythmia, recent myocardial infarct, or enlarged left atrium
- *Computed tomography:* (see also Chapter 30).

The computed tomography (CT) scan is useful in separating hemorrhagic (intracerebral or subarachnoid hemorrhage) from nonhemorrhagic (thrombotic or embolic) stroke. Blood present in a fresh hemorrhage produces an area of increased density; infarction produces an area of decreased density. In addition, the CT scan may help to define the location and size of the abnormality, e.g., vascular territory, superficial or deep location, small or extensive tissue involvement.

1. The CT scan is positive in virtually all cases of *intracerebral hemorrhage (increased density)* and often shows interhemispheric blood or bleeding into brain parenchyma in subarachnoid hemorrhage. These changes are evident within the first hour after onset of symptoms. With the advent of CT scanning, many patients with the clinical diagnosis of thrombosis have been found to have intracerebral hemorrhage.
2. The CT scan is positive in most cases of *cerebral infarction* (*decreased density*), but these changes may only be evident 24

to 48 hours after the onset of symptoms. With contrast enhancement infarcts may mimic tumors on CT scan, but the enhancement is generally not associated with the significant mass effect that occurs with enhancement of brain tumors. In some instances, a mass effect may be present with infarction, raising the question of a brain tumor; MRI, serial CT scans and clinical observation will clarify the diagnosis.

3. A *hemorrhagic infarct* is often secondary to a large embolus. This produces increased density on CT scan. Anti-coagulation should be delayed when hemorrhage is associated with embolic infarction.

4. *Brainstem* hemorrhage may be visible on CT scan, but brainstem infarction usually is not.

5. The CT scan identifies major *shifts of intracranial contents* that may require aggressive medical and surgical measures to control edema (see Chapter 27).

6. *Subdural hematomas* may be recognized on CT scan by shifts of intracranial contents, partial obliteration of a lateral ventricle or of sulci, and changes in density (depending on the age of the lesion) on the surface of the brain.

7. *Brain tumors* are identified on CT scan by characteristic density patterns, contrast enhancement, and mass effects. A small percentage of brain tumors present clinically as strokes.

Magnetic Resonance Imaging

Magnetic resonance imaging (MRI) is playing an increasing role in diagnosis of stroke because:

1. MRI often reveals cerebral ischemia in its early stages, before being visible on CT and often when the CT scan remains negative.

2. MRI will frequently reveal brainstem, cerebellar, or temporal lobe infarcts not visible on CT scan.

3. MRI is more accurate than CT scan in its ability to detect venous thrombosis as a cause of infarction.

4. MRI is more sensitive in detecting small infarcts (e.g., lacunes). The CT scan remains preferable to MRI in the acute stroke patient when hemorrhage is a consideration and when patient cooperation is a problem.

5. Contrast-enhanced MRI may be useful in establishing the age of an infarct and detecting tumor or AVM as a cause for stroke.

NOTE: Single photon emission computed tomography (SPECT) scan may localize ischemia within hours of the event.

Arteriography

Arteriography, either by conventional or digital method, is performed (*a*) to identify surgically correctable lesions (e.g., intracranial aneurysms and arteriovenous malformations, carotid artery stenosis, and ulcerated carotid plaques), (*b*) to clarify an uncertain diagnosis, and (*c*) sometimes when anticoagulation is planned to be more certain of the diagnosis. In guiding arteriography it is important to decide clinically whether disease is in the carotid or vertebrobasilar system. Wherever possible, angiography should be done by selective catheterization techniques by an experienced radiologist.

Electroencephalogram

The electroencephalogram (EEG) may help to localize cortical and sometimes thalamic deficits. It may be abnormal in the early hours after stroke when CT scan remains normal. It is usually normal in posterior-circulation strokes or lacunar (small-vessel) disease and abnormal in anterior-circulation large-vessel disease or with emboli.

EEG is usually abnormal with large-vessel disease or emboli.

It is important to do an EEG if seizure activity is suspected. Weakness after stroke may be due in part to postictal (Todd's) paralysis.

Lumbar Puncture

If the cerebrospinal fluid (CSF) is bloody (greater than 1,000 red blood cells) and the pressure is elevated (greater than 200 mm H_2), the lumbar puncture (LP) supports hemorrhage. Remember, about 10% of intracerebral hemorrhages show no cells in the CSF and a normal pressure. All subarachnoid hemorrhages show grossly bloody CSF, usually greater than 25,000 cells.

A lumbar puncture with 50 to 500 red blood cells (RBCs) is suggestive of embolus, though in the majority of emboli the CSF is clear.

No cells are the expected finding in thrombosis and lacunes. Interestingly, white blood cells (WBCs) may sometimes be seen in the CSF after thrombosis or hemorrhage. Large numbers of red cells (10,000 to 20,000) are occasionally seen after a hemorrhagic infarct secondary to an embolus. With the advent of CT scan, lumbar punctures are infrequently performed in the evaluation of the stroke patient. An LP (see Chapter 29) is performed when:

- Infection is suspected.
- Subarachnoid hemorrhage is a diagnostic possibility. CT scans may be false negative in 5% to 10% of subarachnoid hemorrhage patients.
- Intracerebral hemorrhage is a diagnostic possibility, a CT scan (see above) is not readily available, and there are no signs of increased intracranial pressure.
- Before beginning anticoagulation to rule out bleeding, particularly if CT scan is not available.
- Arteritis is suspected.
- Diagnosis is not clear.

TREATMENT

Cardiac Emboli

Anticoagulation

1. *Anticoagulation* is beneficial in preventing further embolization in patients with cardiac emboli (unless the source is bacterial endocarditis). Thus, diagnosing an embolus of cardiac origin is crucial. It is important to perform a CT scan or MRI to rule out bleeding before beginning anticoagulation. An LP may be done, but it is less sensitive than a CT scan in demonstrating intracerebral hemorrhage and carries the risk of spinal hematoma in anticoagulated patients. The timing of anticoagulation after embolism remains controversial.

Some physicians anticoagulate immediately; others wait 48 hours; still others wait 10 to 14 days if the neurologic deficit is massive to avoid converting a pale infarct into a hemorrhagic one. We feel that the weight of evidence favors immediate anticoagulation if hemorrhage has been excluded and the infarct is small or moderate in size. Particular caution and delay in anticoagulation are advised in elderly patients and in those with massive infarcts (greater than 5 cm) and uncontrolled hypertension. Begin with heparin, then switch to warfarin. Recent data suggests that prothrombin times lower than the traditional 1.5 − control may be adequate for stroke prevention. If the embolus is due to a mural thrombus associated with an MI, anticoagulation is usually continued for 6 months. Anticoagulation for 3 to 6 months is sometimes given for emboli of probable cardiac origin, even though a definite cardiac source cannot be found. If atrial fibrillation and/or rheumatic valvular disease is the cause, long-term anticoagulation is indicated.

Transient Ischemic Attacks

Anticoagulants

2. Some studies on *transient ischemic attacks* have shown a statistically significant reduction of TIAs and subsequent strokes in patients treated with *anticoagulants.* However, most studies did not distinguish those patients with large- or small-vessel disease, or those with TIAs in the anterior or posterior circulation, and arteriography was not carried out in all instances. There are few bleeding complications when the prothrombin time is well controlled, and when high-risk anticoagulant patients are excluded. It appears that there is a beneficial effect of anticoagulants in patients with "stroke in evolution." We believe that anticoagulation benefits patients with a severely narrowed but nonoccluded large blood vessel. For those who have an ulcerated or irregular plaque without severe stenosis that may form the nidus of embolic material we favor antiplatelet agents (e.g., aspirin or ticlopidine). In the patient with TIA in the distribution of a severely stenotic (70–99%) carotid artery, the evidence now clearly favors endarterectomy where angiography and

endarterectomy can be done with low combined morbidity and mortality (less than 3%). We feel anticoagulation is not likely to benefit patients with small-vessel disease, a completed stroke, or a completely occluded large vessel.

3. At the present time, we still favor a minor modification of the Mayo Clinic guidelines (Mayo Clin Proc 1978;53:665) for the management of transient ischemic attacks (assuming that mimickers of TIA, such as migraine and seizures, have been excluded) as follows:

- The majority of patients with vertebrobasilar TIAs are treated medically.
- If a skilled surgeon and an experienced angiographer are available, patients with typical carotid TIAs who are suitable medical risks should have angiography followed by carotid endarterectomy if an appropriate lesion (e.g., greater than 70% stenosis) is found.
- Nonoperated patients with TIAs (due to large-vessel occlusive disease) of less than 2 months' duration are treated with 3 months of warfarin therapy (unless contraindicated) before treatment with aspirin or ticlopidine is begun.
- Nonoperated patients with continuing TIAs of 2 or more months' duration are treated with aspirin or ticlopidine unless there has been a recent increase in the frequency, duration, or severity of TIAs. Under these circumstances, warfarin therapy is advised for 3 months before aspirin is started. Aspirin or ticlopidine therapy should be continued until the patient has been free of TIAs for 1 year.
- No treatment is advised for nonoperated patients whose last episode of TIA was longer than 12 months ago.

Platelet-inhibiting Drugs

4. *Platelet-inhibiting drugs,* such as aspirin, dipyridamole, sulfin-pyrazone, and ticlopidine have been evaluated for treatment of transient ischemic attacks and are used by many physicians. The Food and Drug Administration has concluded that aspirin is effective in reducing the risk of recurrent TIAs. Ongoing studies suggest that ticlopidine may be supe-

rior to aspirin although it is expensive and has more side effects. It is used in patients who have recurrent symptoms on aspirin. As noted above, we follow the Mayo Clinic guidelines for treatment of TIAs. In patients who are not candidates for surgery or anticoagulation or who have TIAs secondary to small-vessel disease, we use aspirin. Clearly, the definitive statement on optimal treatment of transient ischemic attacks in men and women has not yet been made; however there is favorable evidence that aspirin is of value in stroke prevention when given to patients with TIAs.

5. *Lowering markedly elevated blood pressure* in patients with acute stroke may be beneficial when hemorrhage is present but can lead to catastrophic results in the face of thrombosis or embolism, especially if the blood pressure is lowered precipitously.

6. *Surgery* probably benefits the following patients:
   - Those with marked unilateral stenosis of one carotid who have suffered a mild or transient neurologic deficit in that territory (endarterectomy). See results of the North American Symptomatic Carotid Endarterectomy Trial (NASCET). Studies are underway to determine whether surgery benefits symptomatic patients with moderate stenosis.
   - Patients with cerebellar hemorrhage or cerebellar infarction with brainstem compression. Surgery in this group may be lifesaving.
   - Nondominant putaminal hemorrhages that form a large clot and/or cause herniation. Evacuation relieves pressure and prevents brainstem compression.
   - Although controversial, surgery may benefit patients with asymptomatic, severe carotid stenosis. National cooperative studies are currently under way to help determine the role of carotid endarterectomy in carotid stenosis.

   Surgery of the carotid artery is not of benefit in complete carotid occlusion or stroke in evolution. The attempt to improve collateral cerebral circulation by an extracranial-intracranial bypass operation has been studied and found to be of no value.

7. Agents that *reduce increased intracranial pressure* (see Chapter 27) may benefit patients with large strokes associated with

major shifts of intracranial contents during the initial stages of their illness. Intracranial pressure monitoring is performed for these patients in some centers.

8. *Cerebral vasodilators* (CO_2, papaverine) are probably of no benefit.

Subarachnoid Hemorrhage

9. Treatment of *subarachnoid hemorrhage* (SAH) due to aneurysm includes strict bed rest, control of blood pressure, careful medical management including electrolyte monitoring, stool softeners, analgesia, and, whenever possible, surgical ligation or clipping of the aneurysm. Without appropriate treatment approximately 50% of those patients with SAH who survive the first 24 hours, will die within the next 2 weeks. The clinical condition of the patient, the presence of arterial spasm, and the location of the aneurysm influence surgical intervention. Antifibrinolytic agents (e.g., amin-ocaproic acid) had been given to help prevent rebleeding (they act on systemic fibrinolysins) but are falling out of favor because of an increase in ischemic complications. Nimodipine (a "calcium antagonist") may help reduce cerebral arterial spasm. Vasospasm (narrowing of blood vessels on arteriography plus neurologic symptoms) usually begins 3 to 14 days after the initial bleed. There is an increasing tendency for "early" aneurysm surgery following subarachnoid hemorrhage followed by volume expansion in an attempt to prevent rebleeding *and* reduce vasospasm. This approach has had encouraging results at several centers.

RECOVERY

10. A comprehensive *rehabilitation* program that begins in the hospital with physical, occupational, and speech therapy clearly benefits stroke patients. Studies have shown functional gains from such a program that could not be attributed to spontaneous recovery. Likewise, an estimate of the cost-to-benefit ratio showed that the reduced cost resulting from returning patients to the family or to independent living more than paid for the cost of providing rehabilitation services.

11. In atypical nonatherosclerotic stroke, the treatment depends on proper diagnosis and treatment of the underlying disease (e.g., treatment of vasculitis with steroids).

FUTURE

12. The utility of calcium channel blockers in acute stroke is under study.
13. Thrombolytic therapy for embolic and thrombotic stroke has been tried with mixed results. However newer clot-specific agents are being developed and may play a role in stroke therapy in the future.
14. Efforts are under way in some communities to prevent stroke by reducing such risk factors as hypertension, cigarette smoking, and dietary cholesterol, and by early detection of the stroke-prone patient (e.g., those with TIAs).

Suggested Readings

Barnaby W. Stroke intervention. Emerg Med Clin North Am 1990;8(2).

Barnett HJM, Hachinski V. Cerebral ischemia: treatment and prevention. Neurol Clin 1992;10(1).

Biller J. Cerebrovascular disorders in the 1990s. Clin Geriatr Med 1991;7(3).

Brott T. Thrombolytic therapy for stroke. Cerebrovasc Brain Metab Rev 1991;3:91–113.

Caplan LR, et al. Transcranial Doppler ultrasound: present status. Neurology 1990;40:696.

Cerebral Embolism Study Group: Cardioembolic stroke, early anticoagulation and brain hemorrhage. Arch Intern Med 1987;147:636.

Cerebral Embolism Task Force: Cardiogenic brain embolism. Arch Neurol 1986;43:71.

Cromwell RM. Management of subarachnoid hemorrhage. Semin Neurol 1989;9(3):210–217.

Day AL, Salcman M. Subarachnoid hemorrhage. Am Fam Physician 1989;40:99–105.

Estol C, Caplan LR. Therapy of acute stroke. Clin Neuropharmacol 1990;13(2):91–120.

Hart R, Kanter M. Hematologic disorders and ischemic stroke. A selective review. Stroke 1990;21:1111–1121.

Hart RG, Miller VT. Cerebral infarction in young adults: a practical approach. Stroke 1983;14:110.

Lechat P, et al. Prevalence of patent foramen ovale in patients with stroke. N Engl J Med 1988;318:1148.

Lowenstein DH, et al. Acute neurologic and psychiatric complications associated with cocaine use. Am J Med 1987;83:841.

Mohr JP. Lacunes. Stroke 1982;13:3.

North American Symptomatic Carotid Endarterectomy Trial. Beneficial effect of carotid endarterectomy in symptomatic patients with high grade carotid stenosis. N Engl J Med 1991;325:445–453.

Petty GW, Wiebers DO, et al. Transcranial Doppler ultrasonography: clinical applications in cerebrovascular disease. Mayo Clin Proc 1990;65:1350–1364.

Solomon RA, Fink ME. Current strategies for the management of aneurysmal subarachnoid hemorrhage. Arch Neurol 1987;44:769.

Chapter 6

Selected Stroke Syndromes

Lacunes are vascular lesions in the brain commonly seen in hypertensive patients. They are tiny areas of thrombotic infarction that become kernel-sized holes pathologically. It is important to recognize lacunar strokes, because they represent small vessel disease and generally require limited investigation. Control of hypertension, hyperglycemia, and hyperlipidemia, cessation of smoking, and use of antiplatelet agents are likely to improve outcome and prevent future strokes. Look for these characteristic syndromes:

1. *Pure motor hemiplegia.* Lesion in the pons or internal capsule. Paralysis of face, arm, and leg without sensory loss. A right hemiplegia of lacunar origin has no accompanying aphasia; with a left hemiplegia, there are no parietal lobe findings.
2. *Pure sensory stroke.* Lesion most often in the thalamus. Sensory loss in face, arm, and leg, with no hemiplegia or other signs.
3. *Clumsy-hand dysarthria.* Lesion in the pons or internal capsule. Slurred speech with clumsiness and mild weakness of one arm.
4. *Crural (leg) paresis and ataxia (ataxic hemiparesis).* Lesion in the pons or internal capsule. Ataxia and weakness of one leg.

Pure motor hemiplegia is the easiest to recognize; it occurs frequently.

INTRACEREBRAL HEMORRHAGE

CT scan is diagnostic in acute intracerebral hemorrhage.

NOTE: CT may miss hemorrhage in the brainstem and cerebellum due to bony artifacts. If the CT is "normal" and a clinical suspicion of posterior circulation hemorrhage remains, an MRI scan should be obtained.

Bleeding into the cerebellum:

1. Cerebellar hemorrhage is very important to diagnose because it can lead to rapid death via brainstem compression; treatment is surgical evacuation of the clot.
2. Headache, vomiting, and inability to walk with normal lower extremity strength are cardinal features.
3. Strength and sensation are usually normal (unless brainstem compression occurs).
4. The patient may have trouble looking to the side of the lesion (gaze paresis).
5. Nystagmus and limb ataxia are only occasionally present.
6. Ipsilateral facial weakness may be present.
7. Cerebellar infarction with subsequent swelling may mimic cerebellar hemorrhage and require surgical treatment.

Most intracerebral hemorrhage occur in the *putamen.* Look for:

- Hemiplegia
- Striking eye deviation to side of hemorrhage and away from the hemiplegia (Fig. 6.1).
- Headache and often a field defect.
- Cortical deficits, which develop as the hemorrhage progresses.

Surgical evacuation of the hematoma may be useful in nondominant hemisphere cases, particularly if the patient's condition deteriorates. Monitoring intracranial pressure is playing an increasing role in management. Control of blood pressure is important.

In *thalamic* hemorrhage, the patient:

- May or may not have hemiplegia.

Right putaminal hemorrhage

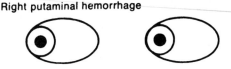

Eyes deviate to the side of the lesion.
Pupils: normal size and reactive.
(seen also with large hemisphere infarcts)

Thalamic hemorrhage

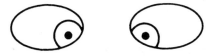

Eyes look down at the nose; vertical gaze is
impaired. Pupils: small and nonreactive.

Pontine hemorrhage

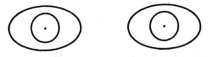

Eyes are midposition with no movement to doll's
eyes maneuver. There may be ocular bobbing.
Pupils: pinpoint, react to light if viewed with a
magnifying glass.

Cerebellar hemorrhage

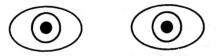

Patient has difficulty looking to the side of the
lesion. There may be skew deviation or a sixth
nerve palsy. Pupils: normal size and reactive.

Figure 6.1. Eye signs of intracerebral hemorrhage. (From Fisher CM.
Some neuro-ophthalmological observations. J Neurol Neurosurg Psychiatry 1967;30:383.)

- Has eyes that look down at the nose, with small and nonreactive pupils (Fig. 6.1).
- Has marked sensory loss.
- Supportive treatment is the only modality available.

Hemorrhage in the *pons* is usually fatal:

- Patient is comatose with small pinpoint pupils (Fig. 6.1.).
- Pupils react to bright light when viewed with a magnifying glass.
- Quadriparesis with up-going toes.
- No horizontal extraocular movements with passive head turning or use of ice water calorics.

NOTE: The most common causes of intracerebral hemorrhage are hypertension and trauma. Other causes include blood dyscrasias, side effects of anticoagulant therapy, drug abuse (cocaine), amyloid angiopathy, brain tumors, and cryptic arteriovenous malformations.

SUBARACHNOID HEMORRHAGE

Subarachnoid hemorrhage classically presents with the sudden onset of severe headache during activity, altered level of consciousness (at times coma), nuchal rigidity, and bloody CSF. There may be autonomic disturbances such as vomiting, fever, and ECG changes. Up to 40% of patients with ruptured aneurysms experience a warning before the catastrophic bleeding. There are usually no focal signs, unless the hemorrhage is into the brain substance or arterial spasm exists. Hemorrhage into the brain substance appears as an increased density on CT scan; arterial spasm generally produces no changes on CT scan. Delayed deterioration in patients with subarachnoid hemorrhage may be due to hydrocephalus, seizures, cerebral edema, vasospasm, or rebleeding.

The most common locations for aneurysms are at various arterial junction points around the circle of Willis at the base of the brain:

1. Posterior communicating artery: may have associated third nerve palsy.

2. Anterior communicating complex: frontal lobe dysfunction may be present.
3. Middle cerebral artery: aphasia or nondominant hemisphere findings.
4. Less common locations include ophthalmic artery (unilateral blindness), cavernous sinus (ophthalmoplegia), and basilar artery (brainstem signs). Arteriovenous malformations (AVMs) may be found anywhere in the brain, but are most common over the convexities. AVMs characteristically present with subarachnoid hemorrhage or with seizures.

NOTE: CT scan is abnormal in 90% of cases of subarachnoid hemorrhage (SAH) and has a false negative rate of 10%. Therefore, do an LP in suspected SAH when CT is "normal."

THROMBOTIC STROKES

The *middle cerebral artery syndrome* is seldom due to thrombosis of the middle cerebral artery; it is usually secondary to an occluded carotid in the neck or an embolus to the middle cerebral. Look for:

- Hemiparesis (greater in face and arm than in leg).
- Aphasia or nondominant hemisphere findings (depending on the side).
- Cortical sensory loss (greater in face and arm than in leg).
- Homonymous hemianopsia.
- Conjugate eye deviation (to the side of the hemisphere lesion).
- "Partial" middle cerebral artery syndromes, almost always of embolic origin, may include (*a*) sensorimotor paresis with little aphasia, (*b*) conduction aphasia, (*c*) Wernicke's aphasia without hemiparesis.

In the *anterior cerebral artery syndrome* look for:

- Paralysis of the lower extremity.
- Cortical sensory loss in leg only.
- Incontinence.

- Grasp and suck reflexes.
- Slowness in mentation with perseveration.
- No hemianopsia or aphasia.
- Left limb apraxia.

Occlusion of the *internal carotid artery* gives a picture resembling occlusion of the middle cerebral artery. When anterior cerebral territory is included in the area of infarction, clinical features of anterior cerebral occlusion also occur. These patients tend to be stuporous or semicomatose due to the large area of infarction usually present.

The *posterior cerebral artery syndrome* presents these features:

- Homonymous hemianopsia (often the only finding); the patient may be unaware of the deficit.
- Little or no paralysis.
- Prominent sensory loss, including to pinprick and touch, may be seen.
- No aphasia or nondominant hemisphere dysfunction.
- Left posterior cerebral artery syndrome patients may show ability to write but not read (alexia without agraphia) and inability to name colors).
- Recent memory loss may be present (involvement of hippocampus) and/or a confusional state initially.

Watershed or *border zone infarction syndromes* (common after anoxia) include proximal arm weakness with distal sparing and transcortical aphasias (see Chapter 4).

Brainstem syndromes never have cortical deficits or visual field defects. One of the most common brainstem syndromes is the *lateral medullary (Wallenberg's) syndrome* caused by occlusion of the vertebral or posterior inferior cerebellar artery (see Fig. 31.6). Look for:

- Ipsilateral to the lesion: facial numbness, limb ataxia, Horner's syndrome (miosis, ptosis, anhidrosis), pain over the eye.
- Contralateral to the lesion: pinprick and temperature loss in arm and leg.
- Vertigo, nausea, hiccups, hoarseness, difficulty swallowing, and diplopia.

If the lesion is typical, treatment is supportive, and these patients usually do well. (Beware of aspiration because of swallowing difficulty.)

Most other brainstem strokes are in the *pons* (see Fig. 31.7).

1. If the lesion is in the *medial* portion of the pons, there is weakness and an internuclear ophthalmoplegia or gaze palsy with little sensory loss.
2. If the lesion is in the *lateral and tegmental* portion of the pons, sensory loss predominates.
3. *Cerebellar signs* are present in lateral lesions and are ipsilateral to the lesion.
4. The *level* of the pons affected is determined by which cranial nerves are involved. The *facial* (seventh) nerve exists from the lower pons and, if involved there, produces ipsilateral total (upper and lower) facial paralysis. If involved higher, there is contralateral facial paralysis that spares the forehead musculature. The *trigeminal (fifth) nerve* exits from the middle of the pons and, if involved at this level, produces ipsilateral loss of corneal reflex and facial sensory loss. The descending tract of the trigeminal (fifth) nerve runs from midpons to lower medulla, and involvement anywhere in its course results in ipsilateral facial pinprick and temperature loss. In *high pontine* lesions, pain and sensory loss are contralateral to the lesion in both face and extremities. In brainstem lesions *below the high pons*, pain and temperature sensations are lost ipsilaterally in the face and contralaterally in the limbs. The cochlear (eighth) nucleus and nerve are in the lower pons and thus ipsilateral deafness and vertigo may accompany pontine lesions.
5. Midbrain strokes frequently involve the third nerve or nucleus and cerebral peduncle, thus producing ipsilateral pupil dilatation, ptosis, ophthalmoparesis, and contralateral hemiplegia (Weber's syndrome) (see Fig. 31.8).

If the deficit in a brainstem stroke is confined to one anatomic area, it generally means that a single branch vessel is involved. If the deficit involves a wider area, the problem may be in the basilar artery itself and catastrophic basilar occlusion may result. Anticoagulation with heparin may prevent the progression from a partial to a complete basilar thrombosis.

NOTE: Rarely, stroke occurs in the spinal cord and presents as paraplegia with urinary retention; a sensory level can usually be found. Vibration and position sense are spared because the cause is often occlusion of the anterior spinal artery in patients with atherosclerotic disease with sparing of the posterior columns. The thoracic cord is most often affected. Treatment is symptomatic, and considerable recovery usually occurs.

Suggested Readings

Barnaby W. Stroke intervention. Emerg Med Clin North Am 1990; 8:267–280.

Pulsinelli W, Levy DE. Cerebrovascular diseases. In: Wyngaarden JB, Smith LH, eds. Cecil's textbook of medicine. Philadelphia: WB Saunders, 1992:ch 468.

Currier RD, Giles CL, DeJong RN. Some comments on Wallenberg's lateral medullary syndrome. Neurology 1961;11:778.

Day AL, Salcman M. Subarachnoid hemorrhage. Am Fam Physician 1989;40:95–105.

Estol C, Caplan LR. Therapy of acute stroke. Clin Neuropharmacol 1990;13:91–120.

Heros RC. Intracranial aneurysms. A review. Minn Med 1990;73:27–32.

Kistler JP, Ropper A, Martin J. Cerebrovascular diseases. In: Wilson JD, Braunwald E, eds. Harrison's principles of internal medicine. New York: McGraw-Hill, 1991:ch 351.

Lehrich JR, Winkler GF, Ojemann RG. Cerebellar infarction with brainstem compression. Arch Neurol 1970;22:490.

Loftus CM. Diagnosis and management of nontraumatic subarachnoid hemorrhage in elderly patients. Clin Geriatr Med 1991;7:569–582.

Mohr JP. Lacunes. Stroke 1982;13:3.

Silver JR, Buxton PH. Spinal stroke. Brain 1974;97:539.

Tsementzis SA. Surgical management of intracerebral hematomas. Neurosurgery 1985;16:562.

Walshe TM, Davis KR, Fisher CM. Thalamic hemorrhage: a computed tomographic–clinical correlation. Neurology 1977;27:217.

Weisberg LA. How to identify and manage brain hemorrhage. Postgrad Med 1990;88:169–175.

Chapter 7

Transient Ischemic Attack

The transient ischemic attack (TIA) is an acute neurologic deficit of vascular origin that clears completely; it usually lasts minutes to an hour, but no more than 24 hours. In some patients, a neurologic deficit related to focal cerebral ischemia persists for more than 24 hours but then clears completely (reversible ischemic neurologic deficit [RIND]). The approach to these patients is similar to that for the patient with TIAs. A TIA is important to recognize because it may be a warning that a more catastrophic and permanent neurologic deficit is imminent. In some instances, treatment is available that will help prevent the impending stroke. One-half to two-thirds of people with thrombotic strokes give a history of a previous TIA, and about one-third of patients with TIAs will go on to have a stroke within 3 years. The symptom complex of TIA represents a variety of pathophysiologic processes, some better understood than others. The following points should be established in the patient with a TIA.

IS THE TIA IN CAROTID OR VERTEBROBASILAR TERRITORY?

The differential points between carotid and vertebrobasilar TIAs were discussed in Chapter 5.

TIAs in *carotid territory* may be associated with stenosis or ulcerative plaques at the carotid bifurcation in the neck. With carotid symptoms, especially in association with a carotid bruit and/or decreased carotid pulse, noninvasive carotid evaluation and/or arteriography are usually performed to define the vascular anatomy and to determine whether the patient is a candidate for carotid endarterectomy (see Chapter 5). Remember, the carotid must have a 75% cross-sectional area reduction before the blood flow is significantly decreased. If the TIA is caused by emboli from an ulcerated plaque, stenosis need not be present. There are patients who have an occluded internal carotid with no symptoms at all. Moreover, patients may have a carotid bruit without stenosis and stenosis without a bruit. There may be an occlusion with a palpable pulse or a decreased pulse in a patent vessel.

TIAs in the *vertebrobasilar territory* are not well understood. The vertebral arteries and their origins have a predilection for atheroma development, and emboli of cardiac origin to the vertebrobasilar territory do occur. Hemodynamic factors may also play a role. Most serious vertebrobasilar disease is intracranial, where surgery is not feasible, and the benefit of operation on the vertebral arteries in the neck is unproven.

In the *subclavian steal syndrome* the patient has a narrowed subclavian artery proximal to the origin of the vertebral artery and the arm "steals" blood from the basilar artery via the vertebral artery. There may be a cervical bruit and a difference in blood pressure between arms. During exercise, the patient may experience symptoms of vertebrobasilar insufficiency. In contrast to other patients with TIAs, those with the subclavian steal syndrome rarely develop a stroke due to the steal, although there may be coexistent serious disease in the carotid arteries.

Vertigo alone is rarely a symptom of vertebrobasilar insufficiency unless other brainstem signs or symptoms are present. Occasionally, an elderly patient may have vertebrobasilar symptoms when turning the head, these being secondary to mechanical factors in the cervical region that reduce blood flow.

IS THE HEART THE SOURCE OF THE TIA?

Emboli from the heart are well-recognized causes of TIAs in both the carotid and vertebrobasilar systems (more common in the carotid) and are seen in rheumatic heart disease, atrial fibrillation, mural thrombus after myocardial infarction, bacterial and marantic endocarditis, atrial myxoma, and with prosthetic valves. Echocardiography is often helpful in diagnosis, especially in patients with known heart disease. Transesophageal echocardiography is proving particularly helpful for detecting cardiac embolic sources such as mural thrombi. Newer techniques, such as "bubble echocardiography," may detect small paradoxical emboli through a patent foramen ovale.

Do not confuse Stokes-Adams attacks with TIAs.

Cardiac arrhythmias may cause TIAs via decreased cardiac output an may require Holter monitoring for identification. Do not confuse Stokes-Adams attacks (syncope due to heart block) with a TIA. Stokes-Adams attacks generally do not have focal neurologic symptoms or signs.

Hypotension may cause focal neurologic symptoms in a patient with compromised cerebral circulation (e.g., due to stenosis of the internal carotid or middle cerebral artery).

TIA: A MIGRAINOUS OR CONVULSIVE PHENOMENON?

Migraine may be accompanied by transient neurologic symptoms or signs (visual disturbances, motor or sensory) and can usually be identified by the headache that follows the neurologic deficit, the gastrointestinal symptoms, and by the fact that it appears in patients younger than those with cerebrovascular disease. Nevertheless, older people do experience migrainous phenomena, and there may not be prominent headache symptoms. Thus, migraine variants in the elderly pose a difficult diagnostic and therapeutic problem. Migrainous sensory symptoms often "march" along an extremity over a period of minutes ("marching numbness").

Keep in mind that *focal seizures* may produce transient neurologic symptoms (numbness, leg or arm movement or weakness) that may persist for hours. Obtain an EEG if seizures are suspected. In addition, *chronic subdural hematoma* and *unruptured cerebral aneurysms* have been reported to present as recurrent transient neurologic deficits.

Some systemic factors may be associated with or mimic TIAs. Well-recognized factors are anemia, polycythemia, thrombocytosis, and hyper- and hypoglycemia, which also may unmask the expression of an old underlying neurologic deficit.

Transient global amnesia (TGA) is a unique syndrome in which, typically, a middle-aged patient suddenly loses recent memory, becomes confused, and asks repeated questions. The patient appears alert, has no motor or sensory signs or symptoms, and retains "personal identity" and the ability to answer questions about job, address, etc. A characteristic feature is the repetition of the same questions by the patient despite being given the answer. The etiology of this dramatic syndrome is unknown, but theories include ischemia involving the hippocampalfornical system, a seizure phenomenon, or a migraine variant. Attacks of TGA are often triggered by special circumstances such as emotional experiences, pain, or sexual intercourse. Attacks usually last hours and clear without residual deficit. These patients often have risk factors for cerebrovascular disease, especially hypertension. Unless attacks are recurrent, treatment, except for risk factors, is usually not necessary.

TREATMENT OF THE PATIENT WITH TIA

After a complete workup (including ECG, possibly Holter monitor or echocardiography, auscultation for bruits, blood pressure check in both arms, noninvasive tests such as ocular pneumoplethysmography, Duplex ultrasound, and sometimes EEG), arteriography may be necessary before deciding on a mode of treatment. To what extent arteriography is indicated depends on the neurologist's and surgeon's evaluations. It is *critical* for the clinician to determine the cause of the transient neurologic deficit (artery to artery embolism, migraine, arrhythmia, etc.) before embarking on a course of therapy.

Recent evidence indicates that endarterectomy is indicated when there is a unilateral severely stenosed (70–99%) carotid in a patient with TIAs in that vessel's territory, if the surgery can be done with less than a 3% morbidity and mortality rate.

Some studies on TIAs and anticoagulation show a statisticaly significant reduction of TIAs and subsequent strokes in anticoagulated patients (see Chapter 5 for discussion of the treatment of TIAs).

A patient is more likely to have a stroke after a few recent TIAs than after TIAs occurring in the distant past. There are a large number of TIAs for which no etiology can be found (e.g., normal cerebral arteriogram and normal cardiac status); this obviously makes the rationale for treatment difficult. Possible explanations include:

- Some TIAs may be associated with small vessel disease not demonstrable on angiography.
- Emboli that result in TIAs may break up as the TIA resolves.
- Some of these episodes are migraine variants.

Patients with TIAs and a negative workup are usually treated with aspirin or ticlopidine.

Suggested Readings

Barnett HJM. Cerebral ischemia and infarction. In: Cecil's textbook of medicine. Philadelphia: WB Saunders, 1988:ch 479.

Dyken ML. Assessment of the role of antiplatelet aggregating agents in transient ischemic attacks, stroke, and death. Stroke 1979;10:602.

Fields WS, Lemak NA. Subclavian steal: review of 168 cases. JAMA 1972;222:1139.

Fisher CM. Migraine accompaniments versus arteriosclerotic ischemia. Trans Am Neurol Assoc 1968;93:211.

Fisher CM. Transient global amnesia. Arch Neurol 1982;39:605.

Grotta JC. Current medical and surgical therapy for cerebrovascular disease. N Engl J Med 1987;317:1505.

Jonas S, Klein I, Dimant J. Importance of Holter monitoring in patients with periodic cerebral symptoms. Ann Neurol 1977;1:470.

Kistler JP, Ropper A, Martin J. Cerebrovascular diseases. In: Harrison's principles of internal medicine. New York: McGraw-Hill, 1987.

North American Symptomatic Carotid Endarterectomy Trial. Beneficial effect of carotid endarterectomy in symptomatic patients with high-grade carotid stenosis. N Engl J Med 1991;325:445–453.

Olsson JE, et al. Anti-coagulant vs anti-platelet therapy as prophylaxis against cerebral infarction in transient ischemic attacks. Stroke 1980;11:4.

Sandercock P. Recent developments in the diagnosis and management of patients with transient ischaemic attacks and minor ischaemic strokes. Q J Med 1991;78(286):101–112.

Sandok B, Furlan A, Whisnant J, et al. Guidelines for the management of transient ischemic attacks. Mayo Clin Proc 1978;53:665.

Toffol GJ. Transient global amnesia. Postgrad Med 1990;88:217–219.

Toole JF, Yuson CP, Janeway R, et al. Transient ischemic attacks: prospective study of 225 patients. Neurology 1978;28:746.

Welsh JE, Tyson GW, Winn HR, et al. Chronic subdural hematoma presenting as transient neurologic deficits. Stroke 1979;10:564.

Chapter 8

Coma

Proper evaluation of the comatose patient usually involves obtaining a history from family and friends, performing a rapid directed physical and neurologic examination, and obtaining certain laboratory studies, while the patient's airway and vital signs are protected. These various parts of the evaluation are often proceeding simultaneously, e.g., one member of the medical team secures the airway, while another talks to the family. An attempt is made to delineate the cause of coma in hopes of finding a treatable process. Treatable causes of coma include metabolic derangements, ingestions, and at times supratentorial processes in the brain (e.g., epidural hematoma). Anatomically, coma implies bilateral hemisphere dysfunction, either structural, drug-induced, or metabolic, unilateral hemisphere disease with compression of brainstem (e.g., epidural hematoma), or brainstem dysfunction (e.g., pontine hemorrhage or compression from a posterior fossa mass). If certain basic points are established when examining the comatose patient, the extent of structural central nervous system (CNS) derangement and the cause usually can be determined. See Table 8.1.

HISTORY

1. Learn from family or friends whether the patient has a pre-existing condition that might explain the coma. Is the patient a diabetic? a drug addict or an alcoholic? Does the patient take sleeping pills? Has the patient been depressed? sustained recent head trauma? had episodes of a similar nature in the past?
2. If a preexisting medical condition exists, is there a factor

Table 8.1.
Coma

States of decreased responsiveness

A. Unresponsive but appears awake (akinetic mutism)
1. Abulic state—frontal lobe disease
2. Psychiatric diseases—e.g., catatonia, hysteria
3. Locked in syndromes—e.g., pontine infarction
4. Nonconvulsive status epilepticus—very rare

B. Decreased responsiveness and appears asleep
1. Drowsiness (light coma)—responds to voice
2 Stupor (moderate coma)—responds to pain
3. Coma (deep coma)—no response
4. Pseudocoma (hysteria)

---

that may have exacerbated it and precipitated the coma (e.g., chronic liver disease and gastrointestinal bleeding; uremia and infection; a seizure disorder and failure to take anticonvulsant medication)?

EXAMINATION

Observe the Patient Carefully

1. Is there decorticate posturing (arm flexion with leg extension), implying hemisphere or diencephalon dysfunction that may be due to destructive lesions or be secondary to a metabolic derangement?
2. Is there decerebrate posturing (extension of legs and arms), implying dysfunction of midbrain or upper pons on a structural or metabolic basis?
3. Is the patient yawning, swallowing, or licking lips? If so, coma cannot be very deep and brainstem function is probably intact.
4. Are there repetitive, multifocal myoclonic jerks or multifocal seizures? These are characteristic of metabolic encephalopathies, such as hypoxia or uremia.

What Is the Respiratory Pattern?

Cheyne-Stokes respiration (a crescendo-decrescendo breathing pattern with apneic pauses in between) implies bilateral hemisphere dysfunction with an intact brainstem. It often accompanies metabolic disorders and congestive heart failure. Rarely, it may be the first sign of transtentorial herniation.

Central neurogenic hyperventilation (rapid deep breathing) usually indicates damage to the brainstem tegmentum between midbrain and pons.

Apneustic breathing consists of a prolonged inspiratory cramp followed by an expiratory pause and is usually seen in pontine infarction.

Ataxic (irregular or agonal) breathing is usually a preterminal event signifying disruption of medullary centers.

Remember, significant damage to the brainstem is rarely accompanied by a normal breathing pattern.

Coma with hyperventilation frequently signifies a metabolic derangement:

- Metabolic acidosis: diabetes, uremia, lactic acidosis, poisoning
- Respiratory alkalosis: salicylates, hepatic failure.

Coma with hypoventilation frequently implies generalized CNS depression secondary to a drug overdose and occurs in patients with chronic pulmonary disease and CO_2 retention.

Does the Patient Respond to External Stimuli?

1. Apply a noxious stimulus to determine whether the patient is unresponsive. Noxious stimuli may elicit decorticate or decerebrate posturing and thus give a clue to the level of brain damage or dysfunction.
2. Test for voluntary response. Let the patient's hand fall toward his face and see if he resists (a check for malingering).
3. Check for a response of the limbs to pain. Is there a low-level reflex, such as flexion, extension, or adduction? Abduction of shoulder or hip usually indicates a higher level (cortical) response. Withdrawal implies purposeful or voluntary behavior.

Examine the Pupils Carefully

Note the size, equality, and light reaction of the pupils.

1. A metabolic (not structural) lesion is usually present if the

comatose patient has no response to external stimuli, absent doll's eyes and corneal reflexes, and yet preserved pupillary responses. Such cases are often secondary to barbiturate ingestion.

2. Glutethimide (Doriden) ingestion and atropine or scopolamine poisoning give large unreactive pupils that give the false impression of a structural lesion.

3. Normal-sized, reactive pupils imply an intact midbrain. Midbrain damage usually produces dilated pupils that do not react to light but may fluctuate in size.

4. Pontine damage produces pinpoint pupils that react to bright light when viewed with a magnifying glass. Heroin and pilocarpine also produce pinpoint pupils.

5. A unilaterally fixed, dilated pupil is seen with damage to the third nerve and often is a valuable early sign of temporal lobe (uncal) herniation from a supratentorial lesion (see Chapter 26).

Check for Corneal Reflexes and Doll's Eyes

Absence of corneal reflexes and doll's eyes usually means pontine damage or dysfunction. If there is no doll's eye response, use ice water irrigation (20 ml in each ear), a strong stimulus of the oculovestibular reflex pathway (be sure there is no wax in the ears and check one ear at a time). Tonically deviated eyes to the side of the irrigation, a normal response, signifies that some brainstem function is intact. An intact cortex (e.g., in "coma" due to hysteria) will cause nystagmus with the fast component opposite to the side of ice water irrigation. Absence of the oculovestibular response implies severe depression of brainstem function. Make sure there is no cervical spine fracture before performing the doll's eye test.

Motor System Examination Is Important

Hyperreflexia and *up-going* toes or hemiplegia usually mean a structural CNS lesion is the cause of coma. Some exceptions are hepatic coma, hypoglycemia, and uremia, which may be associated with focal signs or hyperreflexia. Nonetheless, these should be quickly diagnosed by laboratory studies. *Hyporeflexia* and down-going toes with no hemiplegia generally mean there is no structural CNS lesion, indicating drug ingestion or another metabolic cause.

Other Physical Findings

Careful physical examination may detect other clues to the cause of coma, for example, signs of head trauma in epidural hematoma, barrel chest in pulmonary failure, hepatomegaly in hepatic coma, feeble pulse and hypotension in cardiogenic shock, and stiff neck in meningitis or subarachnoid hemorrhage. There may be cyanosis with hypoxia or "cherry red" appearance in carbon monoxide poisoning. Hypothermia may be associated with barbiturate or ethanol ingestion, while hyperthermia may occur in heat stroke.

LABORATORY STUDIES

Laboratory studies must be carried out to exclude metabolic causes of coma such as hypoglycemia, hypercapnia, hypercalcemia, uremia, hepatic failure, electrolyte disturbance, or toxin ingestion. When clinically appropriate, a CT scan is indicated to rule out intracranial hemorrhage (subdural, epidural, or intracerebral). An EEG is helpful if seizures are suspected; it is also useful for metabolic encephalopathy (slowing) or for psychogenic coma (normal EEG). A lumbar puncture may be needed to detect infection or subarachnoid hemorrhage, although one must be certain that there is no shift of midline structures prior to the lumbar puncture.

Hypoglycemia is one of the most treatable causes of coma.

Remember: Hypoglycemia is one of the most treatable causes of coma. After drawing a blood glucose, give all comatose patients 50 gm of glucose intravenously. If there is a possibility of malnutrition, give 100 mg of thiamine concurrently to prevent Wernicke's encephalopathy. Naloxone (0.4–0.8 mg) should be given intravenously if narcotic overdosage is a possibility. Other therapeutic measures, such as treatment of increased intracranial pressure or gastric lavage after ingestions, may be required.

NOTE: A discussion of the approach to the patient who is "brain dead" or who is thought to be in "irreversible coma" is beyond the scope of this manual (see references by Black at end of chapter). Principles found useful for house officers when approaching the latter problems include (*a*) obtaining appropriate consultations and tests (e.g., EEG) before major therapeutic decisions are made; (*b*) meticulous attention to good communication between all members of the health care team and with family members; (*c*) identification of one physician (usually the admitting physician or primary treating physician) who assumes the primary responsibility for collating the clinical information, consulting with the family, and making the major therapeutic decisions. There are usually "brain death" criteria published at each hospital.

Suggested Readings

Black PMcL, Zervas N. Declaration of brain death in neurosurgical and neurological practice. Neurosurgery 1984;15:170.

Caronna JJ, Simon RP. The comatose patient: a diagnostic approach and treatment. Int Anesthesiol Clin 1979;17:3.

Emanuel E. A review of the ethical and legal aspects of terminating medical care. Am J Med 1988;84:291.

Fisher CM. The neurological examination of the comatose patient. Acta Neurol Scand 1969;45[suppl36]:56.

Levy DE, Caronna JJ. Predicting outcome from hypoxic-ischemic coma. JAMA 1985;253:1420.

Levy DE. Prognosis in non-traumatic coma. Ann Intern Med 1981; 94:293.

Plum F, Posner J. Diagnosis of stupor and coma. 3rd ed. Philadelphia: FA Davis, 1982.

Spudis EV. The persistent vegetative state—1990. J Neurol Sci 1991; 102:128–136.

Chapter 9

Headache

Critical to the evaluation of the patient with headache is obtaining a careful history.

CHARACTER OF HEADACHE PAIN

Migraine headaches are periodic, throbbing, severe, frequently unilateral, and often over the eye(s). Photophobia and sensitivity to sound are common, as are nausea and vomiting.

Tension headaches tend to be diffuse, steady, occipital or frontal, and "band-like," or like a "tight hat."

Headaches associated with increased intracranial pressure or *tumor* are usually not excruciating like migraine.

Cluster headaches are very painful, knife-like, unilateral, and over the eye.

Subarachnoid hemorrhage often is associated with the sudden onset of severe headache ("worst headache of my life") with or without transient impairment of consciousness.

HOW LONG HAS THE HEADACHE BEEN PRESENT?

Migraine usually starts during teenage years (although it may begin at any age), decreases during the 30s and 40s, and may be exacerbated or relieved during menstruation, pregnancy, or around menopause. There is frequently a family history of migraine or childhood motion sickness.

Cluster headaches are usually seen in patients 20 to 60 years old. The headaches come in clusters, last weeks to months, and then subside. Males are more often affected than females.

Tension headaches are usually seen after age 10, are most prominent at times of stress and at the end of the day, and usually do not occur in a cyclic pattern.

Headache that slowly increases in intensity and frequency, does not fit the classic pattern of migraine, tension, or cluster, and appears in someone who has never had headaches before is highly suspicious for *tumor* or raised intracranial pressure.

IS THERE A VISUAL OR OTHER PRODROME?

Migraine may be classic or common.

Migraine may either be *classic* (preceded by visual or other aura) or *common* (no aura). The latter has the same character as classic migraine, but often develops with no warning or builds up slowly.

Classic migraine (migraine with aura) usually begins with a visual prodrome such as flashing lights, blind spots, or hemianopsia. Headache begins when the visual prodrome (usually lasts minutes) is over or subsiding. Other prodromal symptoms may occur with one symptom leading to another— e.g., hemianopsia to difficulty talking, to tingling of face or extremities, to actual hemiparesis ("hemiplegic migraine"). Sensory symptoms that spread slowly along an extremity frequently occur ("marching symptoms"). Classic migraine often has "positive" symptoms followed by "negative" ones—e.g., flashing lights followed by darkness, tingling followed by numbness.

Nausea and vomiting are prominent features of migraine— thus the designation "*sick headaches.*" The gastrointestinal disturbance usually occurs after the headache has been established. Scalp tenderness is also characteristic.

Eye tearing, facial flushing, and stuffy or runny nose, autonomic phenomena associated with *cluster* headache, occur ipsilateral to the headache. Horner's syndrome may be seen.

WHEN DO THE HEADACHES OCCUR?

Tension headaches usually appear toward the end of the day, particularly when the day has been stressful.

Migraine may occur at any time, including times of stress, or may awaken the patient from sleep. It may begin during a "relaxed time"—e.g., on a weekend or vacation, or when a stressful period has ended. Migraine may be associated with menstrual periods or brought on by hunger (skipped meals), alcohol (wine) ingestion, eating chocolate or a hot dog, or at high altitudes. Birth control pills, hyperlipidemia, and hypertension may exacerbate migraine.

Cluster headaches may have the unique feature of occurring at the same time every day. Patients can "set their watches" by the headaches. Cluster headaches, like migraine, may be strong enough to wake a patient and are often precipitated by alcohol ingestion.

WHAT FACTORS MAKE THE HEADACHE BETTER OR WORSE?

Migraine, once established, usually is relieved by sleep and often improves after vomiting.

Sleep has no effect on cluster headache.

Tension headaches are often relieved by relaxation techniques or by massaging the back of the neck.

Headache caused by *tumor* is often made worse by coughing or by straining during a bowel movement (also seen in migraine) and may be at its worst when the patient arises in the morning.

DOES MEDICATION AFFECT THE HEADACHE?

Tension headaches usually respond to aspirin or acetaminophen.

Ergot given early in the course of *migraine* often prevents or alleviates the headaches; some believe this is diagnostic of migraine.

Cluster headaches are helped little by medication once the headache appears. Ergot may be useful, and nasal oxygen may abort the headache.

HOW LONG DOES THE HEADACHE LAST?

Cluster headache lasts minutes to a few hours.

Migraine usually lasts hours to a full day, occasionally longer. Tension headache may become superimposed, prolonging the headache episode ("mixed headache").

Tension headaches usually last hours but can last days.

IS DEPRESSION A FACTOR?

Depression and anxiety are frequently significant factors. Be certain to understand the patient's lifestyle, personality, etc. This is especially important with a patient who has had headaches "every day" for a prolonged time. Explore such issues as adjustment to school or job, domestic strife, illness at home, or recent death.

The vast majority of headache sufferers have a benign or easily treatable cause. Signals of an ominous cause include: headache beginning during exertion, headache accompanied by fever and/or stiff neck, headache in a drowsy or confused patient.

EXAMINATION OF THE PATIENT WITH HEADACHE

Examination sometimes offers clues to the type of headache or to the presence of organic processes, especially if the patient is symptomatic during the examination.

1. Look carefully for focal signs indicative of tumor or other structural lesion (be sure to visualize the fundi).
2. Check for signs of *autonomic dysfunction* during the headache if cluster is suspected—e.g., miotic pupil, ptosis, red eye, tearing, unilateral nasal congestion.
3. Note "sweaty" hands and feet or scalp tenderness (migraine).
4. If the patient develops a stiff neck during the "worst headache of my life," suspect subarachnoid hemorrhage.
5. Patients with *arteriovenous malformations* may present with migraine; be suspicious if migraine attacks are always on the same side. Listen for bruits over the skull or eyes. Migraine that has occurred on either side is usually benign.
6. Headache over the eye in an older person (50 to 70 years of age) may be due to *temporal arteritis.* Check for a tender temporal artery; the sedimentation rate should be elevated. Remember that temporal arteritis can lead to blindness, which can be prevented by steroids.

Temporal arteritis and glaucoma may present as headache in the elderly and may lead to blindness.

7. Note hypertension, which may exacerbate migraine or tension headaches, particularly if the hypertension is labile.
8. Glaucoma is a cause of headache in the elderly; headache, eye pain, red eye, and vomiting are common. Palpate the globe and perform tonometry if glaucoma is suspected. Treatment with pilocarpine or eye surgery may prevent blindness; thus, early diagnosis is crucial.
9. Constant headache in an obese female may be due to pseudotumor cerebri. It is associated with papilledema due to increased intracranial pressure (see Chapter 26).
10. Occipital headache may be due to cervical arthritis, especially in the elderly. Exacerbation of pain by neck movement is helpful in the diagnosis.

Laboratory Studies

Laboratory testing in the patient with headache depends on the clinical impression after obtaining the history and performing a careful examination. All headache sufferers probably deserve a complete blood count, chemistry screen, and sedimentation rate. Beyond that, individualize. Thus:

1. If the history suggests tension headache and the examination is normal, a treatment trial without further testing is reasonable.
2. Most patients with common or classic migraine deserve a CT scan or MRI, at least once for reassurance that another process (e.g., arteriovenous malformation, infarcts due to migraine) is not being overlooked.
3. A CT scan or MRI is mandatory in any patient with focal neurologic signs or signs of increased intracranial pressure.
4. An electroencephalogram (EEG) is often helpful as a noninvasive adjunctive study for focal brain lesions, subdural hematoma, or metabolic encephalopathy. It may be abnormal in migraine.
5. Additional specific studies in patients with headache depend on the clinically suspected etiology—e.g., serum lead level in a car mechanic with headache or arterial blood gases in a patient with chronic lung disease and headache, looking for elevated pCO_2.

TREATMENT TIPS

Migraine

Treatment of the acute headache:

1. *Aspirin or acetaminophen:* May help but usually has been tried by patients by the time they see a doctor.
2. *Fiorinal:* Is often of benefit but may be habit forming when used frequently. Also withdrawal can lead to a caffeine withdrawal headache (Fiorinal contains caffeine).
3. *Ergot* (various preparations are listed under ergotamine tartrate in the *Physicians' Desk Reference*): Effective in prevention or amelioration of headache if given during the prodrome. In some patients, rectal or sublingual preparations may be more effective than oral administration. Once the headache is established, strong analgesia and/or medication to induce sleep may be needed. Ergot derivatives are contraindicated in hemiplegic migraine and in patients with known coronary vasospasm or peripheral vascular disease.
4. *Sumatriptin* a recently introduced 5-hydroxytryptamine receptor agonist appears to be very useful in aborting a migraine headache. It decreases the nausea and vomiting as well, and appears to have few side effects.
5. Never use narcotics for any chronic headache condition.

Prophylactic Medication

1. *Propranolol* is useful for migraine prophylaxis (20 to 40 mg four times a day). Long acting preparations are available. Many feel that selective beta-blockers, such as nadolol, are more effective and have fewer side effects. Use with great caution in patients with asthma, diabetes, and heart disease.
2. *Amitriptyline* is useful for migraine prophylaxis. Begin with 25 to 50 mg at bedtime; 100 to 200 mg at bedtime may be needed before an effect is seen.
3. *Calcium channel blockers* have been useful in prophylaxis, e.g., verapamil, 80 mg three times a day, or long-acting agents.
4. *Methysergide* (Sansert): Given prophylactically to those with frequent incapacitating migraine who have not responded to other medication. It is prescribed daily but not for more than 5 months at a time; the latter precaution reduces such

complications as retroperitoneal fibrosis. It may be restarted after a 1-month hiatus.

5. *Prophylactic phenobarbital* or *phenytoin:* Phenobarbital is useful in juvenile migraine. Either may be useful in adults; phenytoin may be particularly useful in patients with paroxysmal EEG patterns.

6. *Diuretics:* Helpful if the migraine appears to come in association with menstruation. Give 3 to 5 days before the menstrual period starts (e.g., acetazolamide, 250 mg three times a day).

7. *Antihistamines* may benefit some patients with migraine, especially when associated with nasal congestion. Cypro-heptadine (Periactin) has been found particularly useful in juvenile migraine.

8. Nonsteroidal antiinflammatory medications, such as indo-methacin, can provide relief for some patients. They may be of particular benefit if given prophylactically to patients with exertional headache. They are also useful in menstrual-associated migraines (Naprosyn).

NOTE: Avoid factors that precipitate migraine, e.g., alcohol, skipped meals, birth control pills, food containing tyramine or monosodium glutamate. Many patients benefit from regular daily exercise.

Cluster Headaches

1. Cluster headache may be refractory to treatment once the headache is established. Nasal oxygen may abort the headache and sublingual or parenteral ergot is often helpful.

2. To prevent headache once the cluster series has begun, ergot at bedtime or every 12 hours (suppository or intramuscularly), methysergide, lithium carbonate, cyproheptadine, propranolol, chlorpromazine, and prednisone have been found useful.

3. In chronic cluster headache, indomethacin and lithium have been shown to be effective.

Tension Headache

- Aspirin, Fiorinal, acetaminophen.
- Narcotics should not be given for tension headache.

- Tranquilizers.
- Neck massage and heat.
- Relaxation techniques.

Headache Associated with Depression

Antidepressants may relieve headache in certain instances; psychotherapy may be necessary.

Suggested Readings

Caviness VS, O'Brien P. Current concepts: Headache. N Engl J Med 1980;302:446.

Dalessio DJ. Wolff's headache and other head pain. 4th ed. New York: Oxford University Press, 1987.

Diamond S, ed. Headache. Med Clin North America 75(3). Philadelphia: WB Saunders, 1991.

Diamond S, Dalessio D. The practicing physician's approach to headaches. Baltimore: Williams & Wilkins, 1986.

Diamond S, Millstein E. Current concepts of migraine therapy. J Clin Pharmacol 1988;28:193.

Edmerds J. The worst headache ever: ominous and inominous causes. Postgrad Med 1989;86:93–104,107–110.

Hier DB. Headache. In: Samuels M, ed. Manual of neurological therapeutics. Boston: Little, Brown & Co, 1986:15–29.

Jacobson AL, Donlon WC, eds. Head and facial pain. Otolaryngol Clin North Am 1989;22(6), Philadelphia: WB Saunders, 1989.

Mathew NT, ed. Headache. Neurologic Clinics 8(4), Philadelphia: WB Saunders, 1990.

Peroutka SJ. Sumatriptin in acute migraine: pharmacology and review of world experience. Headache 1990;30(2):554–560.

Chapter 10

Dementia

Dementia is a loss of intellectual ability that interferes with a person's ability to function at work or in a social situation.

The goal of the physician is to characterize the patient's dementia in search of a treatable cause.

WHAT IS THE NATURE OF THE DEMENTIA?

Obtain a Careful History from the Family

1. When did difficulties first begin (very important) and how rapidly have they progressed—e.g., did minor problems occur at work?
2. Has the patient been ataxic and/or incontinent (normal pressure hydrocephalus)?
3. Is there a history of getting lost?
4. Has there been a misuse of words (e.g., dysphasia of Alzheimer's disease)?
5. Has the patient become sloppy in habits or dress?
6. Is the patient friendly, or have anger and belligerence developed with the onset of mental difficulties? Has there been a personality change?
7. Has there been toxin exposure (e.g., at work) or alcohol or drug abuse?
8. Is there a history of head trauma before difficulties began? Does the patient complain of headache?
9. Does the patient have an underlying medical illness?
10. Is there a family history of dementia (Huntington's disease, familial Alzheimer's)?

11. Is there a history of strokes or hypertension (multiinfarct dementia)?
12. Have there been symptoms of depression (pseudodementia)?

Define the Mental Status

1. Check the *state of consciousness*. If the patient is not fully awake, one should suspect a metabolic disorder or a space-occupying lesion. Clues that the process may be *delirium* rather than dementia include inattention, fluctuating symptoms, disturbances in sleep, prominent perceptual abnormalities, and increased autonomic activity.

2. Check for *orientation* to place, person, and time. Check for *attention* by digit span or by having patient recite months of the year backwards. If a patient is inattentive, it is difficult to interpret the rest of the mental status examination.

3. Is the patient *aphasic* (see Chapter 4)? Test ability to read a newspaper and write to dictation. If so, were there errors?

4. *New memory:* Can the patient recall three or four unrelated objects after 5 minutes? Remember money placed under the pillow or in a pajama pocket? Test knowledge of recent current events.

5. *Old memory:* Can the patient give correct information about events that occurred some years ago (e.g., naming of presidents)?

6. *Calculation:* Give a simple problem—e.g., six rolls cost $0.12 each; if you give the baker $1.00, how much change would you receive?

7. *Abstraction:* How are a ball and an orange alike? What do a bath tub and the ocean have in common?

8. *Judgment:* What would the patient do upon spotting a fire in a theater or finding a stamped, addressed envelope in the street?

9. *Pictures:* How well can the patient interpret a picture in a magazine? Is there focus on one tiny part; an inability to integrate it (visual agnosia)? Can the patient draw or copy designs (constructional apraxia)?

10. What is the patient's *mood* and *mental content*? Sad or inappropriately cheerful? Fearful or paranoid? Active or apathetic, personally neat or sloppy? Is the patient affect labile?

Perform Careful General and Neurologic Examinations

1. General examination: Is there evidence of liver, kidney, lung, heart, or thyroid disease?
2. Check blood pressure and for evidence of arrhythmia.
3. Are there focal signs, such as a field defect or aphasia? Is there papilledema?
4. Check for pathologic reflexes (e.g., Babinski, suck, snout, grasp).
5. Test for smell. Make certain the patient can hear.

DO THE HISTORY AND PHYSICAL SUGGEST A TREATABLE CAUSE?
Is There a Tumor?

1. Tumors presenting silently as dementia are often in the frontal lobe. Frontal lobe reflexes (suck, snout, grasp) may be present, and there is a "slowness" in carrying out tasks. Smell may be impaired. Tumors occurring in other areas usually give focal signs.
2. Tumors obstructing the third or fourth ventricle may cause hydrocephalus and subsequent dementia, often with few focal signs. Intermittent exacerbation of symptoms is common due to obstruction of CSF pathway.
3. Memory difficulties or language problems are not common early features of brain tumors.
4. The patient with dementia secondary to brain tumor usually presents within 6 to 12 months of the onset of symptoms. (See Chapter 21 for signs and symptoms of brain tumor.)
5. A normal CT scan, with and without contrast, is usually sufficient to rule out tumor. MRI is more sensitive than CT scan for brain tumor, especially for those located in the posterior fossa.

Normal Pressure Hydrocephalus (NPH)

1. Check for memory deficits, ataxia of gait, and incontinence. Lower extremity spasticity and up-going toes are frequent findings. The pathophysiology of NPH is not well understood, but it involves inadequate absorption of CSF over the cerebral hemispheres, leading to hydrocephalus.

A demented patient with a normal gait does not have NPH.

2. Deterioration over 6 to 12 months is usual.
3. NPH may follow subarachnoid hemorrhage, meningitis, or head trauma, but it is often of unknown etiology.
4. If NPH is a serious consideration, CT scan or MRI (and possibly radionuclide cisternography[1]) is indicated. The patients who are most likely to benefit from a shunt procedure are those with a "characteristic" clinical history, a short history of deterioration (6 to 12 months), and abnormal studies.
5. Improvement in gait after LP with removal of 30 ml CSF may be a helpful clue to the diagnosis.

Subdural Hematoma

1. Look for drowsiness in an elderly patient with a recent personality change. Headache is a very important feature and is usually, although not invariably, present.
2. Mental changes usually occur over days to weeks, and sometimes months.
3. There need not be a history of head trauma (absent in one-third of cases).
4. Check for subdural hematoma by performing a CT scan and EEG. Sometimes an isodense lesion will be missed on CT scans. Thus, if the clinical history is suggestive, obtain an MRI even if the CT scan is negative.
5. Bilateral subdural hematoma may appear on CT scan only as bilateral obliteration of cortical sulci; ventricular compression may not be evident. The diagnosis is confirmed by MRI or arteriography.
6. If one suspects subdural hematoma clinically, do not perform a lumbar puncture. It is not diagnostic and may be harmful. (The CSF in patients with subdural hematoma may show xanthochromia and elevated protein, but is normal in about half of proven cases.)

---

[1] Radioactive material injected via LP goes into and stays in the lateral ventricles rather than over the cerebral hemispheres. CT scan or MRI reveals hydrocephalus with essentially normal cerebral sulci. There is controversy as to its value in diagnosis of NPH.

Vitamin B$_{12}$ Deficiency

1. Onset may be insidious over months to years.
2. Although the patient usually has a megaloblastic anemia, the blood smear and neurologic examination may be normal except for the dementia.
3. The EEG is usually abnormal and improves after vitamin B$_{12}$ is given. Neurologic symptoms may precede the anemia.
4. A serum vitamin B$_{12}$ assay is usually a sufficient screening test provided that the patient has not been recently started on vitamins. However, the B$_{12}$ level may be "low normal" in some cases of combined system disease, and therefore a B$_{12}$ bioassay or Shilling test may be necessary for diagnosis.
5. Folate deficiency may produce dementia. Patients who have pernicious anemia treated with folate improve hematologically but progress neurologically.
6. Look for associated paresthesias and posterior and lateral column spinal cord signs (combined system disease, see Chapter 18).

Liver Disease

1. Hepatic dysfunction often presents with defects in memory, abstracting ability, and attentiveness.
2. Mental changes may occur, even though underlying liver disease (such as jaundice) is not apparent.
3. Note somnolence, generalized hyperreflexia, asterixis, myoclonus, and hyperventilation (with respiratory alkalosis).
4. Obtain liver function studies, including an arterial blood ammonia level. Check CSF glutamine and α-ketoglutarate, which are increased in hepatic encephalopathy.
5. Check ceruloplasmin and 24-hour urinary copper levels to rule out Wilson's disease.
6. Consider hemochromatosis.

Depression

Remember, depression may present as dementia and is often termed "pseudodementia." Distinguishing features of pseudodementia include:

1. History of a previous psychiatric disorder is common.
2. Onset can usually be dated, and symptoms are usually of brief duration.
3. Patients complain of cognitive loss yet make little effort to perform even simple tasks; they communicate a strong sense of distress and give frequent "don't know" answers.
4. Associated features of depression may be present, including social withdrawal, ruminations of guilt, apathy, anorexia, weight loss, insomnia, episodes of crying, concentration difficulty, loss of energy, psychomotor retardation, and suicidal thoughts.

NOTE: (*a*) Depression may cause pseudodementia by exacerbating a mild organic dementia. (*b*) Sometimes a trial of antidepressant medication may be worthwhile to exclude depression as a contributing factor.

Other Treatable Causes

Check for syphilis (serologic tests of blood and spinal fluid should be positive), fungal meningitis (CSF pleocytosis, increased protein, and decreased glucose), toxin (metals) or bromide poisoning, uremia, myxedema, Cushing's disease, Wilson's disease, thiamine deficiency, carbon monoxide poisoning, congestive heart failure, drugs such as barbiturates, chronic hypoxia, untreated hypertension, hypercalcemia, carcinoma of the lung, and subacute bacterial endocarditis. All may include dementia in their clinical picture. AIDS patients often develop an encephalopathy with behavioral change and dementia (see Chapter 23).

IS THERE A NONTREATABLE CAUSE?

Alzheimer's Disease

1. The most common cause of dementia is Alzheimer's disease (senile dementia of Alzheimer's type). The pathologic abnormalities when the onset of the dementia is between the ages of 50 and 65 years (previously called presenile dementia) are the same as those found in patients who develop the disease after 65 (senile dementia).

2. Progression is slow over a period of years.
3. Look for memory problems, a tendency to get lost, and language difficulties (dysphasia, word intrusions).
4. There are usually no neurologic signs apart from the dementia; toes are usually down-going, and the patient is generally sociable and neat in the early stages. Later, personality change is frequent. There often is visual agnosia (the ability to see parts of, but not recognize, objects) and motor apraxia (inability to perform certain motor tasks in the absence of paralysis). At advanced stages seizures may occur.
5. Pick's disease resembles Alzheimer's clinically but is very rare. Pathologically it affects frontal and temporal lobes more than parietal lobes.
6. CT scan or MRI usually shows ventricular dilatation and cortical atrophy. EEG shows slowing and irregularity of background rhythms.
7. The pathologic basis of Alzheimer's disease is the subject of much study. There has been major interest in the observed deposition of amyloid beta protein in the brains of Alzheimer patients. Inhibition of this deposition may offer effective treatment in the future.
8. Symptomatic drug treatment involves attempts to improve cognitive function and to improve abnormal behavior. Some of the experimental drugs for the former are intended to augment acetylcholine neurotransmitter functions. Drugs to modify behavior include neuroleptics, anxiolytics and anti-rage medications. Clinical use of these latter medications is described in the articles in Suggested Readings.

Arteriosclerosis (Multiple Strokes)

1. Arteriosclerotic dementia does not mean "getting old"; the term should be reserved for patients with multiple vascular infarcts of the brain (multiinfarct dementia—MID).
2. Look for bilateral pyramidal signs, including up-going toes and a history suggesting previous small focal lesions.
3. Note pseudobulbar signs: emotional lability with easy crying and laughing, increased jaw jerk and gag, dysarthria, and dysphagia.

4. This type of dementia occurs predominantly in inadequately treated hypertensives and is therefore potentially preventable. Treatment of hypertension may prevent progression.
5. CT scan or MRI reveals multiple infarcts.

Creutzfeldt-Jakob Disease

1. The interval between onset and death is usually months.
2. In addition to dementia, patients have upper motor neuron signs, myoclonus, basal ganglia signs, cerebellar signs, startle to noise and bright lights, and characteristic EEG changes (paroxysmal high-voltage bursts).
3. This disease is caused by an as yet unidentified transmissible agent, a prion protein.

Huntington's Chorea

Huntington's chorea presents as insidious intellectual deterioration in association with chorea. Dementia, personality, and emotional disorder may precede the chorea. Inheritance is autosomal dominant. Family history is usually positive, but must be diligently explored. The responsible abnormal gene has been identified and is located on chromosome 4.

Neurodegenerative Disorders

There are several rare childhood neurodegenerative disorders that may present as dementia in adults. These include neuronal intranuclear inclusion disease, Alexander's disease, LaFora's disease, Kuf's disease, and others. The interested reader is referred to the review by Coker.

LABORATORY WORKUP

A basic screen for dementia should include complete blood count, urinalysis, electrolytes, sedimentation rate, vitamin B_{12} and folate levels, liver function tests, calcium, blood urea nitrogen, thyroid function tests, serologic tests for syphilis, human immunodeficiency virus titer (where appropriate), drug levels (where appropriate), ECG, chest x-ray, EEG, CT scan or MRI, LP (if there is no evidence of a mass on the previous studies), particularly if chronic meningitis or opportunistic infection is suspected, and psychologic testing (where appropriate).

With a careful history, physical examination, and the preceding studies, the etiology of dementia should be clear in the vast majority of cases. If the diagnosis remains uncertain, other studies, such as arteriography or brain biopsy, are sometimes necessary. The extent of the workup depends on the patient's age and previous level of function. Remember, the primary goal of the workup of a patient with dementia is to find a treatable cause or a treatable component.

Suggested Readings

Brock CD, Simpson WM. Dementia, depression or grief? The differential diagnosis. Geriatrics 1990;45:37–43.

Coker SB. The diagnosis of childhood neurodegenerative disorders presenting as dementia in adults. Neurology 1991;41:794–798.

Cooper JK. Drug treatment of Alzheimer's disease. Arch Intern Med 1991;151:245–249.

Davidson M, ed. Alzheimer's disease. Psychiatr Clin North Am 1991;14(2).

Elmer M. Management of the behavioral symptoms associated with dementia. Prim Care 1989;16:431–450.

Freedman M, Stuss DT, Gordon M. Assessment of competency: the role of neuro-behavioral deficits. Ann Intern Med 1991;115:203–208.

Gorelick PB, Mangone CA. Vascular dementias in the elderly. Clin Geriatr Med 1991;7:599–615.

Howell T, Watts DT. Behavioral complications of dementia, a clinical approach for the general internist. J Gen Intern Med 1990; 5:431–437.

Kallman H, May HJ. Mental status assessment in the elderly. Prim Care 1989;16:329–348.

Navia BA, Jordon BD, Price RW. The AIDS dementia complex. I. Clinical features. Ann Neurol 1986;19:517.

Tobias CR, Lippmann S, Pary R. Dementia in the elderly. Postgrad Med 1989;86:97–108.

Selkoe DJ. Amyloid protein and Alzheimer's disease. Sci Am 1991;265(November).

Siu AL. Screening for dementia and investigating its causes. Ann Intern Med 1991;115:122–132.

Chapter 11

Seizures

Seizures reflect a disorder of the nervous system due to a sudden, excessive, disorderly discharge of brain neurons.

TYPES OF SEIZURES

Seizures are categorized into two major groups, depending on the source: focal (partial) seizures and generalized (centrencephalic) seizures. In *partial (focal) seizures* (Fig. 11.1A) the initial discharge comes from a focal unilateral area of the brain: temporal lobe, frontal lobe, motor strip, etc. Thus, patients whose seizures begin with their right hands shaking or with an aura of smelling "burned candy" have a partial seizure disorder, attributable to a lesion in the frontal or temporal lobe, respectively. Partial seizures with impairment of consciousness are known as complex partial seizures, to be distinguished from single partial seizures, which have no such impairment of consciousness.

Remember, a seizure can begin focally and then generalize (Fig. 11.1B); this may happen so quickly that it is impossible to see the focality clinically, and the patient can recall no aura. Nonetheless, the EEG usually shows the focality. Partial seizure disorders are usually secondary to local pathology—e.g., trauma, tumor, vascular lesions, or congenital abnormalities.

In *primary generalized seizures* (Fig. 11.1C) the discharge arises from deep midline structures in the brainstem or thalamus. There is no aura, and there are no focal features during the seizure. Examples of primary generalized seizure disorders are petit mal (now called absence) and idiopathic grand mal

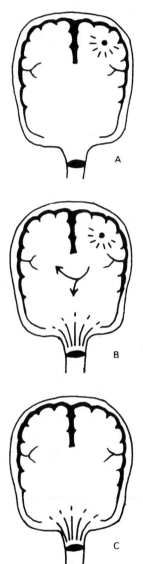

Figure 11.1. Classification of seizure disorders. **A**, Focal seizure. Focal seizure begins from a focal, unilateral part of the cortex (e.g., right-sided tonic movements, eyes deviated to one side, or an automatism of temporal lobe epilepsy). Most seizure disorders are focal, and almost all patients whose seizures begin after the age of 20 have a focal seizure disorder. **B**, Focal seizure with secondary generalization. Focal seizures may activate deep midline structures or spread to the other side, resulting in a bilateral generalized convulsion. The seizure disorder is still classified as focal, even though the focal element may have been transitory before the generalization. (EEG usually shows the focality.) **C**, Primary generalized seizure. No focal component is present either clinically or on EEG. These seizures represent true "idiopathic epilepsy" and usually begin before the age of 20 (e.g., petit mal, grand mal).

of children. A grand mal (now called tonic-clonic) seizure is a major motor seizure involving all extremities and having both tonic and clonic features. It may represent a focal seizure that has spread centrally and generalizes to involve both hemispheres, or it may begin as a generalized seizure from the onset.

Major motor seizures may occur in normal individuals secondary to drug withdrawal or metabolic factors (e.g., uremia, hypoglycemia). These may be focal or nonfocal seizures, and are not believed to represent a true convulsive disorder (see Chapters 24 and 25). Seizures may follow unusual stress ("stress convulsions") and likewise are not considered epilepsy.

ESTABLISH THE "FOCALITY" OR "GENERALITY" OF THE DISORDER
History

1. Exactly how did the seizure start? Find a witness. Did the head and eyes turn? Were there other focal features? Was there an aura?
2. At what age did the seizures begin? This is very important. Primary generalized seizures rarely begin before age 3 or after age 18. "Petit mal" that begins during adulthood is usually a temporal lobe attack.
3. Is there a family history of seizures? This may be present in both types but is more characteristic of generalized seizure disorders.
4. Was there focal trauma at birth or during an accident (head trauma)? Is there a history of a previous neurologic insult (e.g., stroke, encephalitis, meningitis)?
5. Does the patient have abdominal pains, nausea, dizziness, behavioral disturbances, or automatisms (frequent features of temporal lobe epilepsy)? Are there déjà vu phenomena?
6. Is there a history of recent drug or alcohol ingestion or withdrawal?
7. Have there been brief staring spells not followed by postictal confusion or fatigue (absence epilepsy)?
8. Is there an underlying risk factor for seizure present (e.g., HIV infection or diabetes)? Has there been travel to the Southwest or South America (cysticercosis)?

Examination: Search for Focal or Generalized Features

1. Look for postictal paralysis (Todd's paralysis) by checking for asymmetry of reflexes, hemiparesis, up-going toes, or hemiparetic posturing of a foot (everted).
2. Are the eyes tonically deviated during the seizure? For example, a left hemisphere seizure usually drives the eyes to the right.
3. Look for asymmetry of fingernail, toe, and limb size (a clue to early damage of the contralateral hemisphere).
4. Arteriovenous malformations may present as focal seizures; listen for a bruit in any patient with unexplained seizures.
5. Petit mal (a primary generalized seizure disorder of child-hood) can be precipitated by hyperventilation. Have the patient take up to 120 deep breaths and watch for a brief, transient cessation of activity and "glassy stare."
6. Examine the skin carefully. Neurocutaneous disorders, such as neurofibromatosis, tuberous sclerosis, and Sturge-Weber disease, may present with seizures.

Petit mal ppt by hyperventilation

LABORATORY AIDS IN DIAGNOSIS

1. In addition to baseline laboratory studies (including glucose, blood urea nitrogen, calcium, sodium), perform an EEG and an MRI scan or CT scan (MRI is more sensitive in locating the etiology in focal seizures than CT scan) for any unexplained first seizure and an LP if there is any suspicion of infection. If the seizure was focal or if a mass lesion is suspected, be sure there is no papilledema or midline shift before doing the LP.
2. Obtain a sleep-deprived EEG if a temporal lobe seizure disorder is suspected. Frequently, it will bring out the spike focus. In some cases the spike focus can only be seen with special (e.g., nasopharyngeal or sphenoidal) EEG leads.

NOTE: It may be difficult to differentiate between absence and complex partial seizures. Remember that absence seizures have no warning (aura), are abrupt in onset, and are brief (last seconds); the patient has a prompt return to consciousness. Also, absence seizures are characterized by a 3 Hertz spike and wave EEG patttern.

TREATMENT TIPS

Drugs for Focal Seizure Disorders

Carbamazepine (Tegretol) and phenytoin (Dilantin) are the drugs
of first choice used to treat adults with focal (partial) seizures. As a
rule, do not use two drugs unless one drug in adequate dosage
(check blood levels) has failed to control the seizures.

Drugs for Primary Generalized Seizure Disorder

Ethosuximide (Zarontin), valproic acid (Depakene), phenytoin,
phenobarbital, acetazolamide (Diamox), and clonazepam
(Klonopin) are used. Ethosuximide and valproic acid are the
drugs of choice for petit mal. Although primarily for the pediatric patient, ethosuximide and acetazolamide can be beneficial
in the adult who has had primary generalized epilepsy since
childhood or in those with focal seizures and secondary spread.

Status Epilepticus

1. Maintain airway, administer O_2, prevent aspiration, and
   maintain blood pressure. While doing so, obtain a brief history from family or friends and perform a brief examination
   (e.g., is the patient a known epileptic who stopped taking
   medication or developed an infection?).
2. Draw blood to check glucose, electrolytes, calcium, magnesium, complete blood count, and toxic screens. Start an
   intravenous line and administer 100 mg of thiamine followed by 50% glucose.   *Arrival = Doc Statu Epilepticus*
3. *Phenytoin* is an excellent drug for status epilepticus (15
   mg/kg IV over 30 to 45 minutes), and some physicians
   administer it as a first-line drug before diazepam (Valium)
   is used (see below). It works well, it does not depress respiration, and the patient is protected from further seizures.
   Hypotension can occur if the phenytoin is given too quickly.
   Thus, do not administer phenytoin faster than 50 mg/min
   and have blood pressure and ECG monitored periodically
   during intravenous administration. Use cautiously in patients with heart disease. In those with conduction defects,
   phenytoin is relatively contraindicated. For administration,

phenytoin is best given undiluted or intravenously in normal saline; if given in dextrose and water, it will precipitate.

Intravenous Dilantin must be administered in normal saline.

4. *Diazepam* (Valium) (5 mg slowly IV) is also an effective drug to stop seizures. It can be repeated twice at 20- to 30-minute intervals. Diazepam may cause respiratory arrest, especially in patients who have been given barbiturates, and so should be used cautiously. Diazepam may stop seizures, but it does not prevent further seizure activity or stop status epilepticus from beginning again. Thus, after diazepam, administer phenytoin or phenobarbital for continued anticonvulsant control. Lorazepam, a longer-acting benzodiazepine than diazepam, may be used at a dose of 0.1 mg/kg by IV push (use less than 2 mg/min).

5. Sometimes, if diazepam and phenytoin are ineffective in status epilepticus, phenobarbital or paraldehyde may be necessary. If phenobarbital is given after phenytoin, it should be administered cautiously at a dose of 120 mg IM or IV, followed by 120 mg every 30 minutes until 300 to 500 mg have been given. Respiration and blood pressure must be watched carefully, particularly if the patient has received diazepam.

6. Many physicians recommend giving phenytoin followed by phenobarbital for status epilepticus. If this is done, it is then very risky to administer diazepam because of possible respiratory arrest.

7. If the combination of phenytoin and phenobarbital fails to stop status epilepticus, *paraldehyde* (5 ml mixed with 5 ml of mineral oil per rectum, repeated every hour) may be tried to a maximum dose of 15 mg. If this fails, general anesthesia is considered.

8. When it proves difficult to control status epilepticus, there is often an underlying metabolic disorder (e.g., hyponatremia, hypoglycemia) or structural lesion (e.g., subdural, meningitis).

9. The most likely etiology of status epilepticus if there is no prior history is stroke, tumor, or trauma. Otherwise, if there is a prior history of seizures, an intercurrent illness and/or noncompliance with medication is usually responsible.

NOTE: For a hospitalized patient with seizure precautions, have 100% oxygen available at the bedside for use if necessary.

THERAPEUTIC AGENTS

[handwritten: signs toxicity / ① nystagmus ② Ataxia / ↓ the serum / Phenytoin (oral or IV c̄ saline) / >50 = pause value → ↓ myocardial contractility]

Phenytoin

1. The average adult dose is 300 to 400 mg/day. Phenytoin can be given in one daily dose in adults if Dilantin "kapseals," the long-acting form is used, with the patient maintaining blood levels in therapeutic range.

2. Therapeutic blood levels are 10 to 20 μg/ml; levels should be monitored in any patient who has not achieved good seizure control on phenytoin or other anticonvulsants.

3. Administered orally, it takes 4 or 5 days to work; intravenous administration in adequate doses gives therapeutic levels within an hour. Patients may also be given loading doses orally, e.g., 500 mg twice a day, followed by daily maintenance doses. Intramuscular phenytoin is not absorbed evenly, causes muscle necrosis, and should be avoided.

4. Nystagmus on lateral gaze is a good clinical sign that the patient is taking the medication. Ataxia of gait and lethargy are common manifestations of toxicity.

5. Phenytoin is metabolized by the liver, so one can usually give regular doses to patients who have renal disease or are in renal failure. It is of value to check the level of free (unbound, active) phenytoin in these patients.

6. A morbilliform rash occurs in about 4% of patients. If this occurs, it is best to stop the phenytoin and choose an alternate anticonvulsant.

7. Other side effects include hirsutism, gingival hypertrophy, megaloblastic anemia, osteomalacia, lymphadenopathy, and lupus-like syndrome. A teratogenic effect of phenytoin has been reported.

8. Warfarin and isoniazid (INH) enhance the action of phenytoin. Chronic administration of barbiturates may decrease blood phenytoin levels. Patients on phenytoin may have factitiously low thyroid function tests.

Phenobarbital

$t_{\frac{1}{2}} = 96 \text{ hrs in adult}$

1. The average adult dose is 60 mg twice a day.
2. Therapeutic blood levels are 15 to 40 μg/ml.
3. Adults may not tolerate phenobarbital well because of its sedative effect, and children may develop cognitive and behavioral abnormalities.

Carbamazepine (Tegretol) $-1 \; t_{\frac{1}{2}} = (2 \text{hrs})$

1. Dosage: 200 mg, three to four times/day (10 to 25 mg/kg).
2. Therapeutic blood levels are 4 to 12 μg/ml.
3. Toxic side effects include leukopenia, hepatic dysfunction, and rashes. A period of reversible leukopenia usually precedes rare agranulocytosis.
4. Carbamazepine is effective for psychomotor seizures (drug of choice) and major motor seizures.
5. Occasionally, carbamazepine may exacerbate absence seizures in patients being treated for primary generalized tonic-clonic seizures.

Valproic Acid (Depakene)

Contra Pregnancy

1. Dosage: 250 mg, three to four times/day (15 mg/kg).
2. Therapeutic blood levels are 50 to 100 μg/ml, although blood levels may correlate poorly with clinical response.
3. Toxic effects include gastrointestinal disturbances and sedation (especially if the dose is built up rapidly), ataxia, liver dysfunction, thrombocytopenia, and pancreatitis.
4. There is evidence of teratogenic effects; this drug should be avoided in pregnant women if possible.
5. Valproic acid is most effective in absence, myoclonic-akinetic seizures and primary generalized epilepsies. It is structurally different than any other antiepileptic drug (a short-chain branched fatty acid).
6. Interactions with other anticonvulsants include increased phenobarbital levels, and increased or decreased phenytoin levels.

Primidone (Mysoline)

1. Dosage: 125 to 250 mg, three to four times/day (10 to 25 mg/kg).
2. Therapeutic blood levels are 5 to 12 μg/ml.
3. Primidone must be introduced by small increments to avoid toxicity (oversedation, behavioral disturbances, and gastrointestinal dysfunction).
4. A portion of primidone is metabolized to phenobarbital; thus, a combination of barbiturates and primidone often leads to oversedation. Diazepam plus primidone may also cause oversedation.
5. Though still useful in the occasional patient, primidone is being used less often because of its side effects and the availability of other more effective drugs.

WHAT ETIOLOGIC FACTORS ARE INVOLVED?

Metabolic factors, such as hypoglycemia, hypocalcemia, or electrolyte imbalance, may play a role at any age. Other "metabolic" causes include uremia, hepatic failure, and hypoxia. Hypothyroidism can worsen a preexisting seizure disorder.

Drug withdrawal is a common cause of seizures in adults (alcohol, barbiturates, and other sedatives). Alcohol withdrawal seizures ("rum fits") occur 12 to 48 hours after the cessation of drinking (see Chapter 25). Alcoholics with posttraumatic epilepsy secondary to frequent falls may have an exacerbation of seizures when intoxicated.

Exacerbation of a known seizure disorder is common. Persons with a controlled seizure disorder who come to the hospital because of a recurrence usually (*a*) have not been taking their medication (draw blood level); (*b*) have been drinking; or (*c*) have an intercurrent infection. Change in lifestyle, emotional stress, menses, or sleep deprivation may also exacerbate seizures. Temporarily increase the medication if seizures occur during a period of intercurrent infection. Reevaluate anyone with a well-controlled seizure disorder that worsens with no apparent cause.

More than half of the cases of *posttraumatic epilepsy* develop during the first year after injury, and more than 80% develop by 4 years.

Subdural hematoma can be associated with seizures and must be considered in an alcoholic with new onset of seizures.

Etiology as related to *age of onset:*

- Infancy and childhood: birth injury, congenital malformations, infections, trauma, metabolic disorders, idiopathic.
- Adolescence: idiopathic, trauma, drug-related.
- Young adult: trauma, alcohol, neoplasm, drug-related, AVM.
- Middle age: neoplasm, alcohol, vascular disease, trauma, AVM.
- Late life (over 65): vascular disease, neoplasm, degenerative.

NOTE: Idiopathic or primary generalized epilepsy is generally apparent by age 18. Seizures beginning after age 18 are usually due to a focal process or metabolic derangement. Neoplasm is of prime concern during all of adult life. After age 65, vascular disease (stroke) is the most common cause of a first seizure.

Remember

1. Check complete blood count periodically in patients on anticonvulsants, especially those on carbamazepine or ethosuximide. Check liver function in patients on valproic acid.
2. Remind seizure patients of driving restrictions (which vary from state to state).
3. Do not stop anticonvulsants abruptly; drugs should be tapered over a period of weeks.
4. Alert patients to side effects of drugs.

NOTE: Surgery is being used more commonly for the treatment of medically intractable epilepsy via the excision of epileptogenic cortex. This therapeutic option is usually considered after two years of appropriate medication trials fail to bring seizures under reasonable control and where a seizure focus is accessible for surgical removal. The results are encouraging. After temporal lobectomy for temporal lobe foci, approximately 60% of patients became seizure free and 80% are either seizure free or have a significant decrease in seizure activity. The interested reader should refer to the review articles below.

Suggested Readings

Blume HW, Schomer DL. Surgical approaches to epilepsy. Annu Rev Med 1988;39:301.

Cascino, GD. Intractable partial epilepsy: evaluation and treatment. Mayo Clin Proc 1990;65:1578–1586.

Dichter MA. The epilepsies and convulsive disorders. In: Wilson JD, Braunwald E, eds. Harrison's principles of internal medicine. New York: McGraw-Hill, 1991:ch 350.

Engel J. Seizures and epilepsy. Philadelphia: FA Davis, 1989.

Holmes GL. How to evaluate the patient after a first seizure. Postgrad Med 1988;83(2):199–209.

Leppik I. Status epilepticus. Neurol Clin 1986;4:633.

Mattson RH. Selection of drugs for the treatment of epilepsy. In Seminé Neurol 1990;10:406–413.

Pellock JM. The classification of childhood seizures and epilepsy syndromes. Neurol Clin 1990;8:619–632.

Spencer SS. Surgical options for uncontrolled epilepsy. Neurol Clin 1986;4:669.

Chapter 12

Vertigo-Dizziness

Vertigo implies the illusory sensation of turning of spinning—either of the patients themselves or of their environment. *Dizziness* is less easily defined as light-headedness, giddiness, or a feeling or uneasiness in the head. Although vertigo may be distinguished from dizziness by demanding that unmistakable whirling or turning be present, these two symptoms often are clinically indistinguishable and may be approached as one entity.

Is the process peripheral, central, or systemic?

The goal of the clinician is to decide whether the cause is *peripheral* (labyrinth, vestibular, or cochlear nerve), *central* (brainstem, cerebellum, or cerebral cortex), or *systemic* (e.g., cardiovascular, metabolic).

A careful history is often helpful in making this distinction.

HISTORY

1. Are the symptoms paroxysmal, and are they related to head position or other precipitating factors?
2. Is there associated nausea, vomiting, headache?
3. Are symptoms of diplopia, dysarthria, numbness present?
4. Is there tinnitus? Deafness?
5. Is there a lapse of awareness (i.e., to suggest seizures)?

EXAMINATION OF THE PATIENT

1. A general *physical* examination should include careful attention to the cardiovascular system (note arrhythmias).

2. Specifically check the ear canal and hearing (listening to a watch tick, the spoken voice, and finger-rubbing screens three basic frequencies).

3. Perform a complete neurologic examination with special attention to cranial nerves, cerebellar function, and the presence of nystagmus (horizontal, vertical, or rotatory).

4. Check for positional vertigo and nystagmus by having the patient go from a sitting to a supine position while quickly turning the head to the side (Bárány maneuver). Note nystagmus, latency of the response, associated vertigo, and fatigability of the response.

5. Caloric testing (minimal ice water caloric test). Patient lies supine with the head elevated 30°. Irrigate each ear with 0.2 ml ice water (use a tuberculin syringe, check one ear at a time). Nystagmus (fast component) is in the direction of the opposite ear and should last about 1 minute. (Formal calorics involve larger amounts of both warm and cold water.) The important point to notice is the symmetry or asymmetry between the response in each ear.

IS THE LESION PERIPHERAL OR CENTRAL?

Peripheral lesions may be associated with deafness and tinnitus (signs of eighth nerve dysfunction); there are no central signs. If caloric testing reproduces the patient's dizziness or there is has a unilaterally decreased caloric response, the lesion is peripheral. Central lesions are defined by central nervous system signs or symptoms (e.g., cerebellar ataxia, cranial nerve abnormalities, diplopia, dysarthria, papilledema). Vertigo of peripheral origin tends to parallel the nystagmus present. In central lesions, there is often marked nystagmus with little or no vertigo; the nystagmus is most prominent on looking toward the side of the lesion, and the fast component of the nystagmus usually changes with looking in different directions. In acute labyrinthine and vestibular nerve disorders, the nystagmus is usually more prominent on looking toward the good ear. In peripheral vestibulopathy, the patient falls toward the side of the lesion and away from the fast component of nystagmus. In central lesions, such as cerebellar infarction, the patient falls toward the side of the lesion and toward the fast component of nystagmus (see Table 12.1).

Table 12.1.
Differentiation of Peripheral vs. Central Nystagmus

	Peripheral	Central
Latency	3–10 seconds	None
Duration	60 seconds	60 seconds
Fatigability	Yes	No
Associated symptoms	Nausea, vomiting	May have none
Vertical nystagmus	Absent	May be present

Vertical nystagmus is a sign of brainstem disease unless the patient is on medications (especially barbiturates). *Positional nystagmus of peripheral origin* usually begins 3–10 seconds after assuming the new head position (viz., latency of the response), is commonly associated with vertigo and nausea, lasts up to 10 seconds, and is fatigable (it becomes harder to elicit the nystagmus after several consecutive tries). *Positional nystagmus of central origin* begins immediately, may last longer than 10 seconds, and is not fatigable; nausea and vertigo are not prominent. *Rotary nystagmus* is generally seen with peripheral lesions.

IS THE LESION PERIPHERAL?

MÉNIÈRES DISEASE ①VERTIGO, ②TINNING, ⑤DEAFNESS

Middle ear disease may involve the labyrinth. Check for otitis or a history of recent ear infection and other abnormalities of the tympanic membrane. Establish whether the patient has been exposed to ototoxic drugs. Remember, excessive wax in the ear can cause dizziness. Symptoms related to middle ear disease may be brought out by pressure applied to the external ear.

Ménière's disease consists of a characteristic triad: vertigo, tinnitus, and deafness. The underlying mechanism probably relates to swelling of the endolymphatic space. Before vertigo appears there may be buildup with tinnitus and "stuffiness"; the attack itself is violent, with nausea and vomiting, sweating, and decreased hearing. Patients often note a "full" feeling on the side of the affected ear. Nystagmus is present only during the attack, and the direction may vary. Ménière's disease occurs in patients between the ages of 30 and 60, is a paroxysmal disorder, and is accompanied by residual tinnitus and hearing loss after multiple attacks. The vertigo is sudden, recurrent, and severe; usually lasts 1 to 2 hours, not seconds or days. Treatment includes bed rest, sedatives, fluids, antihistamines, and antiemetics during the attack; prophylactically, some use diuretics and sodium restriction. Surgical therapy (endolymphatic shunt) is recommended in some chronic cases.

Benign paroxysmal positional vertigo, or episodic vertigo, occurs when the patient turns the head or changes position; it can be reproduced by testing for positional nystagmus (see above). There is no hearing loss, calorics are normal, and the disorder is self-limited. Treatment with meclizine is usually beneficial; the patient should avoid sudden changes in head position.

Acute labyrinthitis may be secondary to bacterial or viral infections. The onset may be sudden, with severe vertigo and gastrointestinal symptoms. The attack is not as short-lived as that of Ménière's disease and lasts 1 to 3 days. There usually is spontaneous nystagmus toward the good ear, hearing may or may not be affected, and calorics are usually normal. Treatment is symptomatic, i.e., bed rest plus meclizine.

Vestibular neuronitis refers to sudden attacks of vertigo and nausea with no auditory signs or symptoms. Caloric testing shows hypofunction of the affected side, which serves to distinguish it from labyrinthitis. Treatment is symptomatic.

Geniculate ganglionitis causes vertigo associated with ear pain and facial paralysis. It may be due to herpes zoster infection (Ramsay Hunt syndrome). Look for periauricular herpes eruption.

Posttraumatic vertigo is common, and damage to the labyrinth is the postulated mechanism, since symptoms are those of peripheral vestibulopathy. The prognosis is good, with symptoms subsiding over a period of weeks.

DOES THE LESION BEGIN PERIPHERALLY AND THEN SPREAD CENTRALLY?

Acoustic neuroma begins from sheath cells of the vestibular portion of the eighth nerve in the internal auditory canal; thus tinnitus, decreased hearing (e.g., trouble hearing on the phone), and dizziness or disequilibrium are early complaints. As the tumor grows into the cerebellopontine angle, cranial nerve dysfunction (loss of corneal reflex, facial weakness) and cerebellar signs become prominent. Diagnosis is not difficult once there is obvious CNS involvement. Because such tumors can be small and confined to the internal auditory canal, a contrast enhanced MRI is the imaging modality of choice. Early recognition depends on considering the diagnosis in patients with dizziness, unsteadiness, and/or symptoms referable to the eighth nerve (tinnitus and decreased hearing) and ordering brainstem auditory evoked potentials (very sensitive) and MRI with special attention to the internal auditory canals (more sensitive than CT scan).

IS THE LESION CENTRAL?

Posterior fossa tumors may cause vertigo or dizziness; look for cerebellar and other brainstem signs. Check for evidence of raised intracranial pressure in patients with "dizzy feelings" by examination of the fundi.

> To establish vertebrobasilar insufficiency, check for brainstem symptoms or signs.

Vascular disease (vertebrobasilar insufficiency) may cause vertigo. To establish that vertebrobasilar insufficiency is the cause, note other brainstem symptoms (diplopia, slurred speech, numbness, trouble swallowing), or signs (cranial nerve dysfunction, motor or sensory loss). Other important points:

1. Dizziness or vertigo alone may be the *first* sign of vertebrobasilar insufficiency, but most patients have accompanying signs or symptoms of brainstem dysfunction within months of the onset of vertigo.
2. The *lateral medullary syndrome* (see Chapter 6) may begin with vertigo.
3. *Cerebellar hemorrhage or infarction* may begin with the acute onset of dizziness, vomiting, inability to walk or stand, and severe headache (see Chapter 6).
4. Patients with the *subclavian steal syndrome* may experience attacks of vertigo (see Chapter 7).
5. If dizziness is accompanied by *eighth nerve dysfunction* only, it is probably not vascular in origin.
6. Vertigo is seldom a feature of carotid artery disease.

Temporal lobe epilepsy is an important cause of dizziness and vertigo. Note a history of staring spells, automatisms, déjà vu, or abdominal pain. Workup for this seizure disorder should include a sleep EEG. Effective treatment is available (anticonvulsants).

Dizziness after _head trauma_ may be nonspecific, benign paroxysmal vertigo, or represent posttraumatic epilepsy.

Basilar migraine may be associated with vertigo and is characterized by symptoms in the basilar artery territory. Check for vertigo, visual disturbances (including scotomata), tinnitus, blackouts, and associated complaints of throbbing occipital headache when the symptoms subside. It usually occurs in young girls. Treatment includes prophylactic phenobarbital, or propranolol.

Check for a history of _diplopia_. Acute difficulty with eye movements may result in dizziness and/or vertigo. _Multiple_ sclerosis may present with dizziness and/or diplopia due to brainstem involvement (see Chapter 15).

IS THE LESION SYSTEMIC?

Important causes to consider are cardiac arrhythmias, carotid sinus syncope, hyper- or hypotension, congestive heart failure, anemia, hypoglycemia, thyroid disease, and a variety of drugs (e.g., ototoxic drugs, especially the aminoglycosides, antihypertensives, salicylates). Patients with multiple sensory deficits, e.g., poor vision and neuropathy, may complain of dizziness (this is seen most commonly in the elderly).

LABORATORY EVALUATION

Laboratory studies that may prove useful in the evaluation of the patient with vertigo/dizziness include (_a_) auditory evoked responses, particularly sensitive for acoustic neuromas; and (_b_) electronystagmography, particularly sensitive for peripheral labyrinthopathies.

DIZZINESS AND/OR VERTIGO WITH NO APPARENT CAUSE

Vertigo can be caused by psychogenic factors or be due to hyperventilation. In a study of a large series of patients who

DIZZINESS ⟹ CHECK HYPERVENTILATION

complained of dizziness, one of the most common causes was hyperventilation.

Occasionally, despite careful evaluation, a patient's dizziness appears to be idiopathic. In these circumstances, symptomatic treatment and careful follow-up of the patient are required.

TREATMENT

Drugs that may be useful in the treatment of dizziness/vertigo include meclizine, other antihistamines, diazepam, and anticholinergics. The patient should also be advised to avoid sudden positional changes. Limiting intake of caffeine, nicotine, alcohol, and salt may be of benefit. In some cases of severe incapacitating vertigo, surgery (such as closure of an endolymphatic fistula) is necessary.

Suggested Readings

Brandt T, Daroff RB. The multisensory physiological and pathological vertigo syndromes. Ann Neurol 1980;7:195.

Brown JJ. A systematic approach to the dizzy patient. Neurol Clin 1990;8:209–224.

Davis EA. Emergency department approach to vertigo. Emerg Med Clin North Am 1987;:211.

Drachman D, Hart C. An approach to the dizzy patient. Neurology 1972;22:323.

Kumar A, Petchenik L. The diagnosis and management of vertigo. Compr Ther 1990;16(12):56–66.

Nelson JR. The minimal ice water caloric test. Neurology 1972;22:323.

Vesterhauge S. Clinical diagnosis of vestibular disorders: a system approach to dizziness. Acta Otolaryngol [Suppl] 1988;460:114–121.

Weiss HD. Dizziness. In: Manual of neurology. Boston: Little, Brown & Co., 1986.

Chapter 13

Sleep Disorders

Sleep disorders are more common than generally realized. Approximately 10 to 15% of the population have sleep-related problems. Early diagnosis and proper treatment depend on alertness to characteristic signs and symptoms by the primary care physician. Most persistent sleep problems are characterized by excessive sleepiness and/or by difficulty initiating or maintaining sleep. Excessive sleepiness or drowsiness during the day may include falling asleep during activities such as eating, driving, or sitting in a class.

In addition to sleepiness, patients with *narcolepsy* have one or more of the following:

1. *Cataplexy*—sudden loss of muscle tone, induced by emotion or sudden stimuli.
2. *Sleep attacks*—uncontrollable attacks of sleep for short periods.
3. *Sleep paralysis*—upon waking or in transition to sleep, the patient is unable to move.
4. *Hypnagogic* or *hypnopompic hallucinations*—false visual or auditory perceptions just before falling asleep or when just awakening.

Patients with the *sleep apnea* syndrome may have the following:

Restless sleep, enuresis, impotence, morning headaches, memory disturbances, learning problems, heavy snoring, and hypertension.

In *insomnia,* the patient cannot fall asleep at night, has difficulty staying asleep, and/or wakes up early. Disturbed nocturnal sleep leads to daytime drowsiness.

Important points to explore in the history include:

1. Does the patient wake up feeling refreshed, even after a short nap? (narcolepsy)
2. Observations by the patient's sleep partner. Is the patient's sleep restless? Are there sudden jerking leg movements ("restless legs")? Are there pauses of more than 10 seconds between breaths? Is there choking, gagging, or snoring (sleep apnea)?
3. Are there symptoms of depression, including poor appetite, early awakening, weight loss, or sadness, suggesting a secondary sleep disorder?
4. Does the patient have chronic renal failure or chronic alcoholism, each of which has been associated with secondary sleep disorders?
5. Are there symptoms of anxiety that are disturbing sleep, or are there other psychiatric abnormalities ("psychiatric insomnia")?
6. A variety of medications may cause secondary insomnia.

Examination of patients with sleep disorders is usually normal. However, special attention should be paid to:

1. Body habitus and neck size—middle-aged patients with sleep apnea frequently are obese men with thick necks. Sometimes enlarged tonsils or other pharyngeal abnormalities can contribute to obstructive sleep apnea.
2. Memory is frequently impaired in patients with sleep apnea.
3. Retro- or micrognathia (jaw abnormalities) predispose to sleep apnea.
4. Stigmata of hypothyroidism or acromegaly.
5. Hypertension and arrhythmias (especially nocturnal) are associated with sleep apnea.

Laboratory studies of patients with sleep disorders depend on the suspected diagnosis:

In narcolepsy a sleep electroencephalogram (EEG) combined with electromyographic (EMG) and electrooculographic (EOG) monitoring is frequently abnormal, showing rapid eye movement (REM) sleep at sleep outset rather than later in the sleep cycle. A multiple sleep latency test (MSLT), which measures the latency between wakefulness and sleep, is usually abnormal.

In suspected sleep apnea a record of the patient's breathing pattern during sleep is necessary. Monitoring O_2, CO_2 exchange by mask, and diaphragmatic motion can help distinguish obstructive from central from mixed types of sleep apnea.

The above studies are best performed in laboratories with particular interest and expertise in sleep disorders.

TREATMENT

1. Weight loss, treatment with respiratory stimulants, tonsillectomy, palatopharyngoplasty, and, if necessary, tracheostomy may be indicated in the treatment of obstructive sleep apnea. Continuous positive airway pressure (CPAP) at night may prove very helpful in treatment and reduces awakenings and daytime sleepiness. Diaphragmatic pacing is used in the central type.
2. Frequent naps and use of stimulant drugs, such as pemoline and methylphenidate, are used in narcolepsy. Tricyclic antidepressants, such as clomipramine, are useful in cataplexy.
3. The treatment of insomnia is difficult and must be tailored to the individual patient. Modalities include:
   - Environmental manipulation (e.g., altering bed time routine, evening exercise, hot baths before sleep)
   - Relaxation techniques
   - Psychotherapy
   - Short-term hypnotic drug use

Other less common sleep disorders include somnambulism (sleep walking), night terrors and nightmares, enuresis, and nocturnal myoclonus.

Additional tips for patients with insomnia: (a) go to sleep at the same time every night and get up at the same time in the morning; (b) reserve bed for sleeping only (i.e., no eating, reading, or tossing/turning); (c) don't eat large meals before bed; (d) don't use alcohol as a hypnotic; (e) if unable to sleep after a fixed amount of time (e.g., 40 min), get up and do something else.

Suggested Readings

Gottlieb GL. Sleep disorders and their management: special considerations in the elderly. Am J Med 1990;88(suppl 3A):295–335.

Gross PT. Evaluation of sleep disorders. Med Clin North Am 1986;70:1349.

Guilleminault C, Dement WC. 235 cases of excessive daytime sleepiness. J Neurol Sci 1977;31:13.

Kales A. Sleep disorders: insomnia, sleepwalking, night terrors, nightmares and enuresis. Ann Intern Med 1987;106:582.

Kales A. Sleep disorders: sleep apnea and narcolepsy. Ann Intern Med 1987;106:434.

Prinz, PN. Geriatrics: Sleep disorders and aging. N Engl J Med 1990;323:520–526.

Chapter 14

Spinal Cord Compression

Acute spinal cord compression is a neurologic emergency. Prognosis is clearly related to the delay between onset of neurologic symptoms and treatment.

CHARACTERISTIC SYMPTOMS

- Back pain
- Paresthesias in legs ("funny feelings", tingling, or numbness)
- Change in urine function (patient urinates more or less frequently)
- Weakness in lower extremities (especially when climbing stairs)
- Constipation

EARLY SIGNS

- Loss of pinprick sensation or a different reaction to pinprick in the lower extremities. The patient may or may not have a sensory "level" to pinprick. There may be a temperature "level" to a cool object or a "sweat" level.
- Position or vibration loss in the feet
- Slight hyperreflexia in the lower extremities as compared with the upper.

NOTE: The toes are often down-going, and reflexes are reduced in early acute cord compression.)

- Tenderness over the spine is a helpful sign in determining the level of the lesion.

LATE SIGNS

- Definite weakness
- Definite hyperreflexia
- Up-going toes
- A sensory level to pinprick, temperature, and/or vibration. It is often helpful to check vibration sense up and down the spine in search of a level. Check for a sweat level.
- Loss of anal sphincter tone; absent abdominal reflexes; absent bulbocavernosus reflex.
- Urinary retention

CAUSES OF SPINAL CORD COMPRESSION

Epidural Compression

- Metastatic tumor (especially from lung and breast); spinal cord compression may be the initial manifestation of malignancy
- Trauma
- Lymphoma
- Multiple myeloma
- Epidural abscess or hematoma
- Cervical or thoracic disc protrusion or spondylosis or spondylolisthesis
- Atlantoaxial subluxation (rheumatoid arthritis)

Extramedullary, Intradural Compression

- Meningioma
- Neurofibroma

Intramedullary Expansion

- Glioma
- Ependymoma
- Arteriovenous malformation

DIAGNOSTIC STEPS

1. Perform a careful neurologic examination; estimate the level of the cord lesion. Check for postvoid urinary residual.
2. Check for primary tumor sites (e.g., careful breast examination, prostate examination, chest x-ray, routine laboratory studies, including complete blood count, uric acid, acid phosphatase, and PSA).
3. Plain films of the spine should be obtained and may reveal (*a*) vertebral collapse or subluxation, (*b*) bony erosion secondary to tumor, or (*c*) calcification (meningioma).
4. Early consultation with a neurologist and/or neurosurgeon and a radiation therapist is needed.
5. An MRI scan of the spine with sagittal cuts through the entire spine and axial cuts through suspicious areas. If the patient cannot tolerate an MRI, a CT myelogram is usually done.
6. Do not perform an LP if cord compression is suspected; CSF will be examined in conjunction with myelography.
7. MRI may miss a small epidural abscess. If there is a high clinical suspicion, obtain a myelogram/CT.

TREATMENT

Treatment depends on the site(s) of cord block and the etiology. Treatment is most effective if instituted early. Modalities include radiotherapy (for such disorders as metastatic breast or prostate cancer or Hodgkin's lymphoma), surgical decompression for solitary radioresistant extradural solid tumors, or a combination of both.

Dexamethasone (10 to 50 mg IV) is usually given immediately (before myelography, MRI, radiotherapy, or surgery) when compression is suspected clinically, because it may help to preserve spinal cord function.

DIFFERENTIAL DIAGNOSIS OF SPINAL CORD COMPRESSION

1. *Transverse myelitis* is characterized by the acute or subacute development of paraplegia or quadriplegia, occasionally asymmetrical, associated with back pain and sensory loss. It

may or may not be related to a preceding viral illness (e.g., mononucleosis). The CSF may show pleocytosis with increased protein and normal sugar. Myelography or MRI is usually necessary to rule out a compressive lesion. Additionally, MRI may show intramedullary pathology such as a plaque of demyelinating disease. Treatment is supportive. Corticosteroids are often used when the etiology is thought to be postinfectious and/or demyelinating, but their value is debated.

2. *Radiation myelopathy* usually occurs 6 months to a year after irradiation to the thoracic area of the spinal cord (e.g., for lymphoma). Onset may be insidious or abrupt and may be limited to paresthesias or progress to actual paralysis. There is no known treatment, and the myelopathy is probably secondary to vascular damage to the spinal cord. MRI or myelography is needed to rule out a compressive lesion. (Occasionally, radiation myelopathy may occur years after therapy.)

3. *Myelopathy* may also be secondary to toxins (e.g., heroin, arsenic), associated with malignancy elsewhere in the body as a remote effect, or secondary to vascular infarction of the spinal cord.

4. *Acute transverse myelopathy* may be due to anterior spinal artery occlusion. Though motor function and pain and temperature appreciation are usually affected, position and vibration sense (posterior column functions) are usually spared, because of the vascular supply of the spinal cord.

Suggested Readings

Bates DW, Reuter JB. Back pain and epidural spinal cord compression. J Gen Intern Med 1988;3:191–197.

Grant R, Papadopoulos SM, Greenberg HS. Metastatic epidural spinal cord compression. Neurol Clin 1991;9:825–842.

Haughton L. MR imaging of the spine. Radiology 1988;166:297.

Oldfield EH, Doppman JL. Spinal arteriovenous malformations. Clin Neurosurg 1988;34:161.

Portenoy RK, Lipton RB, Foley KM. Back pain in the cancer patient Neurology 1987;37:134.

Siegal T. Current considerations in the management of neoplastic spinal cord compression. Spine 1989;14:223–228.

Weissman G. Glucocorticoid treatment for brain metastases and epidural spinal cord compression: A review. J Clin Oncol 1988;6:543.

Chapter 15

Hyperreflexia and Hyporeflexia

Normal reflexes suggest that the motor system between cortex and muscle is functioning normally. Pathologically hyperactive reflexes imply disease between cortex and spinal cord, and hypoactive reflexes imply disease between spinal cord and muscle.

HYPERREFLEXIA

Hyperreflexia signifies an upper motor neuron lesion along the neuraxis from cortex to lateral columns of the spinal cord. When anterior horn cell or peripheral nerve is involved, there is usually hyporeflexia.

> Hyperactive reflexes in the presence of down-going toes are usually normal.

Many people have exaggerated reflexes that may appear hyperactive. A good rule is that symmetrical hyperactive reflexes in the presence of down-going toes are usually normal. If the hyperactive reflexes truly reflect pyramidal tract disease, the toes should also be abnormal. Abdominal reflexes (stroke skin next to umbilicus) may be absent on the side of pyramidal tract dysfunction. Check for a brisk jaw jerk in patients with hyperreflexia; its presence suggests bilateral lesions above the midpons.

A unilaterally up-going toe, or *hyperactive reflexes on one side,* implies damage to one side of the nervous system. Decide whether this represents an old lesion not requiring further investigation or a newly developing one. Check for:

1. History of birth injury. An otherwise normal person may have unilateral hyperreflexia with no apparent cause. This may be due to birth injury with mild cerebral palsy.
2. Old neurologic disease. A patient with a history of meningitis, stroke, subdural hematoma, etc., may have unilateral hyperreflexia. Remember, a small stroke may not have been recognized by the patient.
3. Newly developing signs or symptoms. If history suggests this, a full investigation is warranted.

Bilateral Hyperreflexia

Bilateral hyperreflexia with up-going toes implies bilateral pyramidal tract dysfunction. Note the following:

1. With spinal cord compression look for metastatic disease in the adult, intrinsic tumor in the younger person, or bony abnormalities of the spine, all of which may cause bilateral hyperreflexia. Carefully check for sensory level, sweat level, local back tenderness, and other features of spinal cord compression (Chapter 14).
2. Cervical spondylosis is the most common cause of spinal cord dysfunction in the elderly. Ask about neck pain. Look for bilateral hyperreflexia, muscle wasting in arms and/or hands, decreased range of motion of the neck, and degenerative changes on x-ray of the cervical spine (see Chapter 18).
3. Multiple sclerosis (MS) is an important cause of hyperreflexia in a young person. The reflexes may be markedly increased, and in some instances there may be unilateral hyperreflexia. These patients may not have noticed the transitory episode that caused the hyperreflexia; however, a careful history and examination usually delineate a story suggestive of multiple sclerosis. Patients with MS have "multiple lesions in time and space":
   - MS may take different forms: (a) relapsing, remitting disease. In early stages, patients recover completely from attacks. Later, they may accumulate disability with each attack; (b) chronic progressive disease, usually with progres-

sive spinal cord dysfunction. The progressive form may
evolve from the relapsing form or be progressive from
onset. Although it is difficult to predict the course of an
individual patient, patients with multiple relapses and
accumulating disability or those that enter the progressive phase have the poorest prognosis.

- Common symptoms: unilateral loss of vision that has
resolved (optic neuritis), bladder disturbances (incontinence), sensory symptoms (heaviness or numbness in
an extremity), diplopia, speech and gait difficulties.

- Frequent physical findings: pallor of the optic disc, afferent pupillary defect (Marcus-Gunn pupil) internuclear
ophthalmoplegia, cerebellar ataxia, dysarthria, hyperreflexia, spasticity and weakness of lower extremities.

- Diagnosis is based on history and physical examination
and spinal fluid abnormalities that include increase in
mononuclear cells, elevated gamma globulin, and the
presence of oligoclonal banding. An MRI of the brain is
usually abnormal (periventricular an/or multiple white
matter lesions) and has become a major tool in diagnosing MS. In many instances it has replaced the spinal tap.
Remember, white matter abnormalities may occur with
monophasic illnesses that are not MS and are more frequent in the elderly. At least 75% of MS patients have
abnormal visual evoked responses, even those patients
without visual symptoms. Abnormal visual evoked
responses or MRI abnormalities may establish the diagnosis in a patient with only spinal cord abnormalities by
identifying a "second lesion" in the nervous system.
Abnormalities of T lymphocyte function are found,
especially in chronic progressive disease.

- Treatment is both supportive and directed at underlying
immune abnormalities. Supportive treatment includes
baclofen for spasticity, oxybutynin (Ditropan) for urinary frequency, and amantadine for fatigue. Steroids
are usually given during acute exacerbations and
include oral prednisone and high-dose IV methylprednisolone (1 gm/day over 5–7 days). IV methylprednisolone is recommended for acute optic neuritis, as
oral prednisone may cause worsening in some patients.
Long-term steroid therapy is not recommended.

Accumulating evidence has demonstrated that MS is an immune-mediated disease. Immune suppression slows disease progression in some patients, whereas treatment with gamma interferon (an immune enhancer) exacerbates the disease. Beta interferon has been approved by the FDA for treatment of relapsing-remitting MS. Intermittent pulse therapy (every 4–8 weeks) with IV methylprednisolone or cyclophosphamide as is used in lupus nephritis protocols may help stabilize younger patients with actively progressive disease. Immunosuppresion carries serious potential risks and should be undertaken with caution. Many new clinical trials of immunotherapy are in progress in MS, and patients should contact the National Multiple Sclerosis Society for the latest information.

Remember that spinal cord compression is an important differential diagnosis in the patient with possible multiple sclerosis, and a myelogram or MRI is often performed to rule out surgically correctable lesions.

4. *Multiple small strokes* (état lacunaire) can cause bilateral hyperreflexia and are frequently seen in the elderly patient with hypertension or diabetes. Check for a history of multiple, small cerebrovascular accidents (although they may have been clinically silent) as well as other evidence of vascular disease. Search for other associated signs of "multiple stroke" syndrome: emotional lability, increased jaw jerk, increased gag reflex (features of pseudobulbar palsy), and ataxia. In addition, there is usually dementia with memory impairment (see Chapter 10).
5. *Familial spastic paraplegia* is a cause of hyperreflexia; be sure to check the family history. Also tropical spastic paraparesis is caused by HTLV-1 infection.
6. *Metabolic causes* of hyperreflexia include hepatic and uremic encephalopathy.
7. *Amyotrophic lateral sclerosis* (ALS) causes increased reflexes secondary to pyramidal tract involvement. This may occur in brainstem (increased jaw jerk) and/or spinal cord. In addition, fasciculations and muscle wasting occur due to associated anterior horn cell disease (e.g., fasciculations of

the tongue). The combination of upper and lower motor neuron signs in spinal cord and brainstem without sensory loss is virtually diagnostic of ALS.

8. Hyperreflexia can be seen in otherwise normal anxious patients.

NOTE: Hyperreflexia in both arms and legs implies a lesion at the cervical cord or higher; *hyperreflexia in the legs only* implies a lesion below the cervical cord. There are three exceptions to this basic anatomic rule:

1. *Cerebral palsy.* Leg fibers may be selectively involved in the white matter of the hemispheres, giving increased reflexes in legs only ("spastic diparesis").

2. *Parasagittal intracranial mass.* By virtue of its location, it may affect cortical leg fibers, producing hyperreflexia in legs only, mimicking a cord lesion. Headache, seizures, and/or papilledema may be present.

3. *Hydrocephalus* may present with spastic paraparesis because parasagittal leg fibers are stretched most by dilated lateral ventricles. Arnold-Chiari malformation may be associated with a spastic paraparesis.

HYPOREFLEXIA

Hyporeflexia usually indicates peripheral nerve disease with one component of the reflex pathway being abnormal: peripheral nerve, sensory root, anterior horn cells in cord, motor root, or muscle. Reflexes can be reinforced by having the patient pull his hands apart or bite down when reflexes are tested. Areflexia implies no reflexes, even with reinforcement; reflexes present only with reinforcement imply an intact reflex pathway and may or may not be abnormal. Consider the following points when confronted with hyporeflexia:

- *Normally hypoactive reflexes.* Occasionally one sees otherwise normal individuals with hyporeflexia and no obvious cause.

- *Delayed relaxation phase of the reflex.* This unique "hypoactive" reflex is classic for hypothyroidism and at times serves as the first clue to this metabolic abnormality (it is best seen in the ankle jerk).

- *Spinal shock.* This is a very important cause of areflexia and is often seen during the initial stages of cord damage–whether traumatic, vascular, or neoplastic in orgin. Although compressive damage to spinal cord generally causes hyperactive reflexes, remember that acutely (during the first days, and often as long as 1–2 weeks), reflexes may be depressed or absent. Be sure to check for a sensory level, especially if there is leg weakness.
- *Acute stroke.* Initially, there is usually hyporeflexia on the side of the hemiparesis; later, hyperreflexia develops.
- *Asymptomatic areflexia with a large pupil.* This is a benign syndrome (Adie's), consisting of generalized areflexia plus a large pupil that reacts to accommodation but not to direct light.
- *Myopathy.* Muscle disorders may cause hyporeflexia (although usually not areflexia). Remember, weakness from muscle disease is generally more marked proximally (shoulder and hip), while weakness from peripheral nerve disease is more marked distally (hand and foot).
- *Isolated unilaterally absent reflex.* This very important sign of disc disease compressing spinal roots can be seen with diseases affecting specific peripheral nerves. Some examples are as follows:
    1. *Unilaterally absent ankle jerk* should arouse suspicion of disk disease with compression of the S1 root on the same side. (Ask the patient about sciatic pain and check straight leg raising.) Similarly, but less frequently, the knee jerk may be absent unilaterally with root disease at L3 or L4 or with femoral neuropathy (see Chapter 19).
    2. *Unilaterally absent brachioradialis, biceps, or triceps* reflex may imply impingement on C5, C6, or C7 nerve roots, respectively, in the cervical region from cervical spondylosis.
    3. Remember, *mononeuropathy and plexus injury,* whether traumatic or from tumor, are other important causes of asymmetrical reflex loss (see Chapter 19).

A patient with no reflexes usually has a neuropathy.

Bilateral areflexia is the hallmark of neuropathies, a broad category of diseases affecting peripheral nerves. If one cannot elicit reflexes, the patient usually has a neuropathy. Neuropathies may be categorized into motor and sensory neuropathies, axonal or demyelinating, although there is considerable overlap, and often a "sensorimotor" neuropathy exists.

1. *Areflexia with acute or subacutely developing motor weakness and little sensory loss* is the classic presentation of the *Guillain-Barré* syndrome, or acute inflammatory demyelinating polyneuritis. The patient has tingling or "funny feelings" in the hands and feet, although motor weakness exceeds the sensory symptoms. Inflammatory polyneuritis may begin days to weeks after a systemic infection (usually viral) or immunization, or it can follow such nonspecific factors as a surgical procedure.

   a. *Clinical characteristics.* In the *mild* form the patient's motor difficulties are confined to problems with gait and trouble using the upper extremities. The dysfunction does not progress, and a clue to the diagnosis is the areflexia. The *moderate* form is an extension of the mild form but includes enough weakness that the patient is unable to walk alone. In the *severe* form, the ascending weakness becomes an ascending paralysis that may include respiratory muscles and involve cranial nerves. These patients require tracheostomy and intensive respiratory care. A form where cranial nerve involvement predominates (Miller-Fisher variant) exists. *Autonomic dysfunction* may occur, causing fluctuations in blood pressure, temperature, and heart rate. Rarely patients may die, particularly where autonomic dysfunction and arrhythmias are prominent, but most recover and are able to walk again.

   b. *Diagnosis.* Clinical features include an ascending progressive muscle weakness that is more prominent proximally, *areflexia,* a mild distal sensory loss, and bilateral facial weakness (an important clue). An LP usually shows raised CSF protein with few or no white cells. CSF protein may be normal during the initial stage of the illness but usually rises within a few days. Nerve conduction studies are abnormal early in the course of the disease.

   c. *Treatment.* In Guillain-Barré syndrome, the severity of the paralysis may not be evident at first. Therefore the physician must recognize that he or she is dealing with acute inflammatory polyneuritis and carefully monitor respiratory function, including blood gases and vital capacity, until the paralysis has reached a plateau. This is crucial. The use of steroids is no longer recommended (except in chronic inflammatory demyelinating polyneuropathy). A treatment modality whose efficacy has been established is plasmapheresis. This is of greatest efficacy when begun early in the disease (less than 7 days after onset). IV gamma globulin may also be of benefit in these patients. A mainstay of treatment remains supportive, including meticulous pulmonary and nursing care and treating of autonomic dysfunction, including cardiac arrhythmias. Currently 85–90% of patients make complete recovery, but this may take weeks or months.

d. *Differential diagnosis.* Check for acute intermittent porphyria, tick paralysis, Lyme disease, botulism, polyarteritis, toxin exposure, and diphtheria (palatal and extraocular muscle palsies); these processes may mimic the Guillain-Barré syndrome. Think of polio in unimmunized children. Also, test for mononucleosis, hepatitis, and *Mycoplasma* infection, which may have been the preceding illness. A similar picture with a slower course may represent chronic inflammatory demyelinating polyneuropathy (CIDP).

2. *Areflexia with sensory neuropathy and little or late developing motor loss:*

a. *Diabetes.* Various neuropathies may be associated with diabetes (see Chapter 20); most common is a bilateral symmetrical neuropathy manifested by absent ankle jerks and decreased vibration sense. Motor weakness is minimal.

b. *Alcoholism* (nutritional and toxic deficit). These patients have a sensory neuropathy, often painful, involving feet and hands, including decreased vibration sense (see Chapter 25). They have numbness and tingling, and their feet are very tender to touch. Weakness is minimal, although this distal sensory neuropathy occasionally progresses to an incapacitating motor neuropathy.

   c. *Vitamin B₁₂* deficiency may produce lower limb areflex and distal paresthesias.

   d. *Uremia.* The patient often has "restless legs" and may develop profound distal sensory loss with muscle atrophy, areflexia, and burning sensations (see Chapter 24).

   e. *Tumors* (especially lung). Malignancy may have, as its initial manifestation, a relatively pure sensory neuropathy with numbness, paresthesias, and "sensory" ataxia of hands and feet; motor involvement may appear later. Always be suspicious of occult malignancy with a "remote" effect in the patient with a sensory neuropathy of unknown etiology.

   f. *Amyloid,* often associated with a blood dyscrasia or tumor, can present with a sensory neuropathy with autonomic manifestations.

   g. Infectious causes such as Lyme disease and human immunodeficiency virus may cause a sensory neuropathy. The former usually involves a mixed motor and sensory radiculoneuropathy, or mononeuritis multiplex, while the latter involves a distal symmetrical polyneuropathy or chronic inflammatory demyelinating polyneuropathy.

   h. *NOTE:* A familial sensory radicular neuropathy with autosomal dominant inheritance may present during the second and third decades. Fabry's and Refsum's diseases may present as sensory neuropathy.

3. *Bilateral areflexia and neuropathy on a familial basis.* The prototype for familial neuropathy is *Charcot-Marie-Tooth* disease (peroneal muscular atrophy). These patients have sensory loss, "champagne-bottle" legs, a widespread areflexia not merely confined to the ankles, and pes cavus. Familial neuropathies may be associated with other inherited neurologic diseases, with other symptoms being present–e.g., cerebellar tremor, nystagmus, and ataxia.

4. *Autonomic neuropathy* commonly accompanies diabetes, alcoholism, and Parkinson's disease and may also occur as a primary disease or as a paraneoplastic syndrome. Symptoms include orthostatic hypotension, sweating abnormalities, GI symptoms, impotence, and bladder dysfunction.

WORKUP OF NEUROPATHIES

In most instances, the etiology of a patient's neuropathy can be determined, particularly with intensive evaluation. Check these important points when dealing with a neuropathic process of undetermined cause:

1. Is there evidence of toxin exposure: arsenic (painful red feet, gastrointestinal disturbances), thallium (alopecia), lead (affects upper extremities, including motor neuropathies with wrist-drop, and causes lead line in gums), other metals (copper, zinc, mercury)? Consider organic toxins and occupational exposures. Check for antibodies to GMI and MAG.

2. Check for drugs that may cause neuropathy. Nitrofurantoin, isoniazid, and vincristine are common offenders. Check each medication the patient takes.

3. Does the patient have an associated systemic illness: hypothyroidism, syphilis, amyloid (large tongue, gastrointestinal symptoms), myeloma or other gammopathy, leprosy (anesthetic skin patches), lupus, AIDS, Lyme disease, sarcoid, polyarteritis, pernicious anemia, porphyria, diabetes, renal failure, polyarteritis, rheumatoid arthritis, Sjögren's, systemic sclerosis?

4. Is the neuropathy relapsing? An important group is the chronic inflammatory demyelinating type of poly-neuritis that responds to steroids; other relapsing neuropathies may be due to alcohol ingestion, porphyria, or lead poisoning.

5. Electromyography and nerve conduction studies should be performed when the diagnosis is in doubt; nerve conduction velocities are usually decreased in peripheral neuropathy but may be normal or mildly reduced in axonal neuropathy. Depending on the neuropathy, motor and sensory conductions may be differentially affected, and axonal vs. demyelinating neuropathies may be distinguished.

6. Nerve biopsy is sometimes diagnostic (e.g., with sarcoidosis or amyloid or with vasculitic neuropathy).

7. Spinal fluid in patients with inflammatory neuropathy, diabetic neuropathy, and neuropathies associated with cancer usually shows elevated protein with or without a cellular response.

TREATMENT OF NEUROPATHIES

Removal of the offending agent in toxic neuropathies (e.g., alcohol) and, where possible, treatment of an associated systemic illness (e.g., Lyme disease) are important. Vitamin replacement is indicated in deficiency states. Steroids, and in some instances plasma exchange, are useful for relapsing demyelinating polyneuritis; steroids and cyclophosphamide are useful in polyarteritis.

NOTE: A mnemonic device that may aid in remembering causes of neuropathy is "DAG THERAPIST": **D**iabetes, **A**lcohol, **G**uillain-Barré, **T**oxins, **HE**reditary, **R**efsum's, **A**myloid, **P**orphyria, **I**nfection, **S**ystemic, and **T**umor.

Suggested Readings

Cohen JA, Gross K. Peripheral neuropathy: causes and management in the elderly. Geriatrics 1990;45(2):21–34.

Cohen JA, Gross K. Autonomic neuropathy: clinical presentation and differential diagnosis. Geriatrics 1990;45(7):33–42.

Dyck PJ. Intensive evaluation of referred unclassified neuropathies yields improved diagnosis. Ann Neurol 1981;10:222.

Dyck PJ, Thomas PK, Lambert EH. Peripheral neuropathy. Philadelphia: WB Saunders, 1984.

England JD. Guillain-Barré syndrome. Annu Rev Med 1990;41:1–6.

IFNB Multiple Sclerosis Study Group. Interferon beta-1b is effective in relapsing-remitting multiple sclerosis. I. Clinical results of a multicenter, randomized, double-blind, placebo-controlled trial. Neurology 1993;43:655–661.

McKhann GM. Plasmapheresis and Guillain-Barré syndrome: analysis of prognostic factors and the effect of plasmapheresis. Ann Neurol 1988;23:347.

Weiner HL, Hafler DH. Immunotherapy of multiple sclerosis. Ann Neurol 1988;23:211.

Weiner HL, Mackin GA, Orav EJ, et al. Intermittent cyclophosphamide pulse therapy in progressive multiple sclerosis: final report of the Northeast Cooperative Multiple Sclerosis Treatment Group. Neurology 1993;43:910–918.

Chapter 16

Myopathy

When confronted with a patient who may have a myopathy, the physician must establish whether the weakness is indeed myopathic, if the myopathy is congenital or acquired, and if acquired, whether it represents a manifestation of another illness (e.g., thyroid myopathy).

HISTORY

In a patient complaining of weakness in whom the diagnosis of myopathy is made, one finds:

1. The weakness is *gradual* rather than sudden in onset and is symmetrical.
2. There are no paresthesias or "pins-and-needles" feelings in the limbs.
3. Climbing stairs and combing hair are particularly difficult *(proximal weakness)*.
4. Bowel and bladder function are not affected.
5. The weakness is usually painless.
6. Cramps may be present.

Establish the following points:

1. Is there a *family history* of a similar disorder (e.g., in the muscular dystrophies)?
2. Is there myotonia (inability to release grip)?
3. Is there trouble swallowing (polymyositis), variation in the weakness that occurs during the day, or diplopia (myasthenia)?

Table 16.1.
Myopathic and Related Disorders

Acquired myopathies
- Polymyositis (idiopathic or associated with tumor)
- Thyroid
- Steroid-associated
- Alcoholic

Muscular dystrophies (onset after age 30 is rare)
- Duchenne: affects young boys, death by age 20
- Facioscapulohumeral: autosomal dominant, onset between ages 10 and 20
- Limb-girdle: affects shoulder and pelvis musculature, onset between ages 15 and 25
- Myotonic dystrophy: usually manifests in early adult life with myotonia, peripheral muscle wasting, endocrinopathies, impotence, frontal balding, cataracts; inheritance is autosomal dominant

Myasthenia gravis: classically involves ocular muscles and variability is characteristic; there may be proximal muscle weakness even though it is not a myopathy.

4. What was the exact age of onset? This may help to distinguish congenital and acquired myopathies.

PHYSICAL EXAMINATION

In the myopathic patient:

1. *Proximal limb strength* is more impaired than distal strength (except in myotonic dystrophy). Check deltoids (shoulder) and iliopsoas (hips). Check neck flexion. Weakness tends to be *distal* in neuropathies. Weakness may be proximal in Guillain-Barré syndrome, but there are areflexia, sensory symptoms, and raised CSF protein.
2. *Neck flexion* is much weaker than neck extension.
3. *Reflexes* are preserved or slightly decreased except in late stages of disease.
4. *Sensation* is unimpaired. This is *not* true in neuropathies.

Check these points, which help to distinguish one myopathy from another:

1. Note whether *facial muscles* are involved. Have patient shut eyes tightly, puff cheeks, or attempt to whistle (difficult in facioscapulohumeral).
2. Check for *fatigability,* especially of extraocular movements. Practically all patients with myasthenia gravis have ptosis or diplopia at some time in the course of their illness, and their weakness fluctuates. They may also have dysarthria and dysphagia.
3. See if *pelvic* and *thigh muscles* are more involved than those of the head and shoulders (limb-girdle).
4. Check for *myotonia* by percussing the thenar eminence or the tongue, and check for lid myotonia by having the patient shut the eyes tightly and then quickly open them. Patients with myotonia may be unable to "let go" after handshake.

LABORATORY STUDIES

Characteristic features of myopathies include:

- Elevated muscle enzyme levels, especially CPK. SGOT, aldolase, and LDH may also be elevated.
- Normal spinal fluid, including the protein level.

Special studies usually done on the patient suspected of myopathic disease include:

- Electromyogram (EMG) and nerve conduction study.
- Muscle biopsy

IS THERE A TREATABLE MYOPATHY PRESENT?

Check for the following:

1. *Thyroid myopathy* (both hyper- and hypothyroidism).
2. *Steroid myopathy.* Has the patient been on steroids for another disorder? (Fluorinated steroids are especially prone to causing steroid-induced myopathy.) Does the patient have Cushing's disease?
3. *Idiopathic polymyositis.* There is usually an elevated sedimentation rate and, at times, evidence of other connective tissue disease, such as dermatomyositis, rheumatoid arthritis, or

lupus erythematosus. Treatment is with steroids. In steroid-resistant cases, or when steroid toxicity develops, methotrexate or cyclophosphamide may be effective.

4. *Polymyositis* associated with malignancy. Some adults with polymyositis will have the symptoms as a remote effect of cancer. Polymyositis may also be associated with sarcoid. Look for rash of dermatomyositis.

5. *Alcoholic myopathy.* Check for a history of alcoholism. Does the patient have an associated cardiac myopathy? These patients may have a painful myopathy.

6. *Periodic paralysis.* Attacks are often related to cold, food, or exercise. Check the serum potassium level during an attack. Family history is often positive for a similar disorder. Myotonia is present in the hyperkalemic form.

7. *Polymyalgia rheumatica.* Although this disorder is not associated with muscle weakness, patients complain of muscle and joint aches. The sedimentation rate is elevated, and the disorder is exquisitely responsive to low-dose steroids.

8. *Myasthenia gravis.* Does the patient have fluctuating weakness during the day? The diagnosis of myasthenia is usually confirmed by a Tensilon test, repetitive nerve stimulation and single fiber EMG, or acetylcholine receptor antibody level. Treatment involves use of anticholinesterases, prednisone, thymectomy, and in some cases, immunosuppressive therapy or plasmapheresis. Myasthenia, usually classified with myopathies, is actually a disease of the neuromuscular junction. The etiology relates to a postsynaptic defect of acetylcholine receptors at the neuromuscular junction, caused by circulating antibodies and thymus-derived lymphocytes directed against the acetylcholine receptor. The presence of anti–acetylcholine receptor antibodies in the blood is highly specific for myasthenia gravis, but the level does not correlate with the severity of the disease.

9. *Eaton-Lambert syndrome.* This is a rare neuromuscular junction syndrome seen in association with systemic cancer. Unlike myasthenia, ocular involvement is rare.

NOTE: The gene for Duchenne's muscular dystrophy has been identified, and a protein, dystrophin, appears to play a major role in the disease process.

Suggested Readings

Brooke MH. A clinician's view of neuromuscular diseases. 2nd ed. Baltimore, Williams & Wilkins, 1985.

Drachman DB. Present and future treatment of myasthenia gravis. N Engl J Med 1987;316:743.

Mastaglia FL, Ojeda VJ. Inflammatory myopathies. Parts 1 & 2. Ann Neurol 1985;17:215 & 1985;17:318.

Plotz PH. Current concepts in the idiopathic inflammatory myopathies: polymyositis dermatomyositis and related disorders. Ann Intern Med 1989;111:143–157.

Riggs JE. Muscle disease: neurologic clinics. Philadelphia: WB Saunders, 1988.

Rowland LP. Dystrophin. N Engl J Med 1988;318:1392.

Chapter 17

Tremor

Tremor involves rhythmic oscillating movement of the extremities or head. Types of tremor include: (*a*) action tremor of the essential, familial, or senile type: (*b*) resting tremor associated with Parkinson's disease, (*c*) intention tremor associated with cerebellar dysfunction (e.g., brought out by "finger-to-nose" movement of an extremity). Other disorders of movement are also discussed in this chapter.

ACTION TREMOR

Action tremor is a tremor of posture or activity that disappears at rest; it is usually asymmetrical. Some people may be unable to sign their name in public or lift a cup to their lips because of exacerbation of the tremor with anxiety or use of the arms. Patients may have an associated head tremor, although seldom is there a head tremor without an arm tremor; there may also be an associated vocal tremor; legs are rarely involved. Action tremor is of lower amplitude than parkinsonian tremor and is unaccompanied by the rigidity and the slowness (bradykinesia) of Parkinson's disease. Action tremor may be familial, senile, or "essential" and may be helped temporarily by alcohol ingestion (a diagnostic maneuver). Neurologic examination is otherwise normal in patients with action tremor.

Differential Diagnosis

Action tremor may be associated with pheochromocytoma, hyperthyroidism, toxins, and administration of amphetamines, lithium, and amitriptyline; it is made worse by phenothiazines. Remember, tremor may be associated with Wilson's disease.

Treatment

Propranolol (Inderal), 60–240 mg/day in three or four divided doses, is the drug of choice and is usually effective. Remember, propranolol may be contraindicated in patients with pulmonary or cardiac disease and may cause depression and impotence. Primidone (Mysoline) may be helpful (25–50 mg two or three times a day). Diazepam (Valium), 10–30 mg/day may also be of benefit, especially when given in conjunction with propranolol.

NOTE: Normal persons may have a physiologic tremor that may be periodically enhanced (e.g., by anxiety, drugs).

PARKINSON'S DISEASE

The tremor of Parkinson's disease is a gross, 3–7/second, "pill-rolling" resting tremor that improves with movement. It occurs in the older patient and is not helped by alcohol. Examination usually reveals other features of parkinsonism: decreased facial expression, decreased blinking, limb rigidity, shuffling gait, slowness in movement (bradykinesia), and change in voice. The patient may also be depressed and, in advanced stages, suffers from dementia. The three cardinal features of Parkinson's disease are tremor, bradykinesia, and rigidity. Some include postural instability as a cardinal feature. Parkinson's disease is secondary to a loss of dopamine in the nigrostriatal pathways. This upsets the normal dopaminergic-cholinergic balance. The most effective treatment for moderate to severe Parkinson's disease is exogenous replacement of L-dopa; anticholinergic medication is also of benefit.

Treatment

There are many regimens for the treatment of Parkinson's disease. Most clinicians find that the tremor of Parkinson's disease is helped most by anticholinergic medication, and the akinesia and rigidity by L-dopa.
1.   Patients with mild parkinsonism may be treated with amantadine (Symmetrel), an antiviral agent that probably benefits parkinsonian patients by releasing dopamine from presynaptic storage sites. A response should be seen within a few days. Side effects are few and include nausea, visual halluci-

nations, and livedo reticularis (a venous mottling of the skin, usually around the knees). Livedo reticularis is benign and does not require discontinuation of the drug.

2. Anticholinergic medication, e.g., benztropine mesylate (Cogentin) or trihexyphenidyl (Artane), is particularly useful for tremor. Side effects include dry mouth, blurred vision, urinary retention, and confusion in patients with advanced disease or dementia. Patients with glaucoma should only receive anticholinergics in conjunction with treatment by an ophthalmologist. Antihistamines, e.g., diphenhydramine (Benadryl), may also be tried and are weak antiparkinsonian agents.

3. L-Dopa is usually given in combination with a peripheral dopa decarboxylase inhibitor, carbidopa (Sinemet). Some physicians use L-dopa as the first drug, particularly in those patients whose parkinsonian symptoms interfere in a major way with their functional status. The decarboxylase inhibitor increases the amount of L-dopa reaching the CNS. Thus, it decreases the amount of L-dopa needed, and some of its side effects (e.g., nausea and vomiting) are avoided. Three strengths of Sinemet in scored tablets are available: 10/100 mg, 25/100 mg, and 25/250 mg (carbidopa/L-dopa). A new long-acting form is available with a strength of 50/200. Patients are usually begun on 10/100 mg three times a day and dosage is increased gradually every other day until the desired therapeutic effect is reached or side effects occur. Most patients require 25/250 mg three or four times a day and a minimum of 75 mg of carbidopa for the L-dopa to be effective. The most common side effect of L-dopa therapy is development of chorea (involuntary, "jerk-like" movements that may involve both face and extremities). There may also be dystonia, agitation, hallucinations, and paranoia. This "hyperkinesia" represents the opposite end of the spectrum of bradykinesia and akinesia that are characteristic of parkinsonism and requires lowering the L-dopa dosage. With lowering of dosage, parkinsonian symptoms may recur. At this stage, administration of small amounts of L-dopa alone may be of benefit. Amantadine and anticholinergic drugs can be used concomitantly with L-dopa. Amantadine may be effective in patients receiving L-dopa, even though it did not help when given alone.

4. *Bromocriptine* (usual starting dose is 1.25 mg twice a day, which is then gradually increased), a dopamine agonist, has also been used in the treatment of Parkinson's disease. It may be useful in patients with long-standing Parkinson's disease in whom the effects of L-dopa have worn off. A combination of L-dopa plus bromocriptine is often useful. *Pergolide*, another dopamine agonist, is often used as an alternative to bromocriptine. The mean therapeutic dose is 3 mg/day. Treatment begins with 0.05 mg and is then slowly increased in 0.1–0.25 mg increments.

5. *Deprenyl*, a monoamine oxidase B inhibitor, is commonly used as an adjunct to therapy, as it may delay the progression of Parkinson's disease. It is now used by many as a first-line treatment for early Parkinson's disease.

Note the following:

a. Tricyclic antidepressants can be used for depression in patients receiving L-dopa (they may slow absorption via their anticholinergic effects); monoamine oxidase inhibitors are not recommended.

b. Phenothiazines, haloperidol, and reserpine aggravate parkinsonian symptoms. Clozapine is a new antipsychotic that causes no movement disorder.

c. Pyridoxine antagonizes the effect of L-dopa but not of Sinemet. Remember, pyridoxine is a vitamin and is often found in vitamin pills.

d. α-Methyldopa (Aldomet) may potentiate or antagonize the effects of L-dopa.

e. Other side effects of L-dopa (whether given with or without carbidopa) include postural hypotension (usually asymptomatic) and insomnia.

f. The Shy-Drager syndrome is a progressive neurologic disorder consisting of impotence, postural hypotension, and parkinsonism due to basal ganglia degeneration. L-Dopa is ineffective. Other uncommon neurologic disorders may have symptoms of parkinsonism, including olivopontocerebellar degeneration, progressive supranuclear palsy (paralysis of vertical gaze, neck rigidity) striatonigral degeneration (poor response to L-dopa), and Wilson's disease (liver dysfunction, Kayser-Fleischer ring).

g. Parkinsonism may be secondary to chronic manganese or carbon monoxide intoxication, MPTP (a "designer" drug), or encephalitis (oculogyric crises).

h. Physical therapy with a specific list of home exercises is useful in Parkinson's disease. Patients should be encouraged to remain active and mobile.

i. Some patients report a "wearing off" effect of L-dopa, i.e., 2–3 hours after the previous dose. This is treated by giving medication more frequently and/or adding other antiparkinsonian drugs. Sustained-release Sinemet (Sinemet-CR) has been introduced and may obviate this problem.

j. The "on-off" effect of L-dopa refers to the sudden loss of the therapeutic effect of L-dopa, which can last minutes to hours. The "on-off" effect is poorly understood, and several treatment regimens have been tried, e.g., special diets (especially low-protein diets), discontinuing medication (drug holiday), and use of drugs such as bromocriptine, pergolide, and monoamine oxidase B inhibitors (Deprenyl).

k. Drug-induced parkinsonism, a toxic effect seen in patients receiving high doses of neuroleptic drugs (e.g., phenothiazines), is clinically similar to idiopathic parkinsonism. Treatment includes lowering the dose of the neuroleptic drug plus anticholinergic medication. Remember, anticholinergics plus phenothiazines potentiate the appearance of tardive dyskinesia (see below). L-Dopa is contraindicated in drug-induced parkinsonism because it usually exacerbates the psychosis.

l. An experimental approach to the treatment of Parkinson's disease by transplanting adrenal (dopamine-producing) tissue into the basal ganglia remains under study.

TARDIVE DYSKINESIA

Tardive dyskinesia (TD) develops in a significant number of patients on prolonged treatment with neuroleptic drugs and often persists after the antipsychotic medication is discontinued. Some patients may develop TD after a relatively short (less than 1 year) duration of exposure. The drugs most frequently associated with tardive dyskinesia are the phenothiazines and haloperidol. Clinically, patients develop an oral-buccal-lingual dyskinesia (tongue protrusion, lip smacking, facial grimacing); involuntary movements may involve the limbs and trunk as well. It is felt that tardive dyskinesia is caused by overactivity of brain dopamine associated with denervation hypersensitivity of brain dopamine receptors caused by chronic neuroleptic medication. The main therapeutic approach in tardive dyskinesia is to deplete brain dopamine with drugs such as reserpine. Another approach is to use cholinergic agents such as deanol to modulate the balance between dopamine and acetylcholine in the striatum. Obviously, elimination or reduction of neuroleptic therapy should be carried out. For many patients, tardive dyskinesia is refractory to medical treatment despite the large number of drugs that have been tried in this disorder.

OTHER MOVEMENT DISORDERS

1. *Hemiballismus*, wild, involuntary flinging of an extremity, is often secondary to a cerebrovascular accident affecting the subthalamic nucleus. There also may be hemichorea. Treatment with haloperidol (3–8 mg/day) is usually effective, presumably by blocking "overreactive" dopamine receptors in the striatum. Some investigators have used perphenazine.

2. Acute *dystonic* postures (e.g., turning of the neck) may occur as an idiosyncratic reaction to neuroleptic drugs, such as phenothiazines and prochlorperazine (Compazine), and usually occurs in young adults. They respond dramatically (within minutes) to intravenous administration of diphenhydramine (Benadryl) 75 mg or benztropine mesylate (Cogentin) 2 mg. In addition to acute dystonia and drug-induced parkinsonism (discussed previously), neuroleptics can also cause akathisia (persistent motor restlessness).

3. *Myoclonus*, or shock-like, nonpatterned contraction of a portion of a muscle, an entire muscle, or a group of muscles occurs in a wide variety of disorders, including anoxic brain damage, myoclonic epilepsy, and certain degenerative diseases. It can also be seen in metabolic encephalopathies (particularly uremic) and certain drug intoxications (e.g., imipramine). Drugs that may be useful in treatment include clonazepam, valproic acid, and 5-hydroxytryptophan.

4. *Chorea*, involuntary, irregular, jerky movements of various body parts resembling restlessness; a feature of Huntington's disease, Sydenham's chorea or in association with pregnancy (Chorea gravidarum).
5. *Athetosis*, slow writhing movement of fingers and hands.
6. *Tics*, erratic, rapid, stereotyped, irresistible behaviors; may be associated with sniffing, snorting, and involuntary vocalization (Tourette syndrome).

Suggested Readings

Calne DB, Rinne UK. Controversies in the management of Parkinson's disease. Movement disorders 1986;1:159.

deJong GJ, Meerwaldt JD, Schmidt PIM. Factors that influence the occurrence of response variations in Parkinson's disease. Ann Neurol 1987;22:4.

Findley LJ, Koller WC. Essential tremor: A review. Neurology 1987;37:1194.

Helme RD. Movement disorders. In: Samuels M, ed. Manual of neurology. Boston: Little, Brown & Co, 1991.

Hubble JP, Busenbark KL, Koller WC. Essential tremor. Clin Neuropharmacol 1989;12(6):453–482.

Jankovic J, Fahn S. Physiologic and pathologic tremors. Ann Intern Med 1980;93:460.

Johnson WG, Fahn S. Treatment of vascular hemiballism and hemichorea. Neurology 1977;27:634.

Kang UJ, Burke RE, Fahn S. Natural history and treatment of tardive dystonia. Movement Disorders 1986;1:193.

Klawans HL, Moses H, Nausieda PA, et al. Treatment and prognosis of hemiballismus. N Engl J Med 1976;295:1348.

Koller WC, Huber SJ. Tremor disorders of aging: diagnosis and management. Geriatrics 1989;44(5):33–41.

Parkinson's Study Group. The effect of Deprenyl on the progression of disability in early Parkinson's disease. N Engl J Med 1989;321:1364.

Chapter 18

Ataxia

Ataxia is a disorder of coordination and rhythm. Because many parts of the nervous system participate in carrying out coordinated movements, ataxia may result from anatomic dysfunction at different levels of the neuraxis. The best way to establish the cause of ataxia is to determine what level of the nervous system is involved. In this chapter, ataxia is classified anatomically, and some of the common causes of ataxia are discussed.

IS THE LESION IN THE FRONTAL LOBE?

(Mechanism: involvement of corticocerebellar connections, i.e., frontoponto cerebellar pathway).

1. *Tumor.* Meningioma, glioma, or metastatic tumor may involve the frontal lobes. Patients may have signs of cerebellar disease, i.e., staggering gait, difficulty performing rapid alternating movements, and even nystagmus, although these signs are present in only about half of patients with frontal lobe tumors. Patients with "frontal ataxia" tend to fall backwards. Other features of frontal lobe dysfunction include perseveration, grasp and suck reflexes, incontinence, and slowness in thinking and initiating conversation. There is often headache, and patients may be demented (see Chapter 21). Diagnosis is via CT scan or MRI.
2. *Anterior cerebral artery syndrome.* A thrombotic occlusion of this artery affects the frontal lobes (see Chapter 6). A large aneurysm of the anterior communicating artery may also affect the frontal lobes.
3. *Hydrocephalus.* Enlargement of the frontal horns of the later-

al ventricles affects leg fibers and may produce ataxia. In addition, there is memory loss and incontinence. Hydrocephalus may occur with tumors that obstruct the ventricular system or with more diffuse problems of CSF absorption (e.g., normal pressure hydrocephalus, see Chapter 10).

IS THE LESION *SUBCORTICAL*?

(Mechanism: involvement of corticocerebellar connections plus pyramidal tract dysfunction.)

1. *Multiple strokes* (état lacunaire). In addition to ataxia, there is emotional lability, brisk reflexes including increased jaw jerk, dysarthria, and dementia (see Chapter 10).
2. *Ataxic hemiparesis* is a lacunar syndrome with the lesion in the internal capsule or pons.

IS THE LESION IN THE *BRAINSTEM*?

(Mechanism: involvement of cerebellar tracts.)

1. The two most common causes of ataxia secondary to brainstem lesions are *stroke* and *multiple sclerosis.* Diagnosis is based on history and finding other brainstem signs (e.g., crossed motor or sensory findings, internuclear ophthalmoplegia, nystagmus, dysarthria).

IS THE LESION IN THE *CEREBELLUM*?

(Mechanism: direct involvement of coordination pathways.)

1. *Signs* of cerebellar dysfunction include limb, trunk, gait, and speech ataxia, nystagmus, and hypotonia. Depending on whether midline or lateral cerebellar structures are involved, there may or may not be limb ataxia or prominent lateral gaze nystagmus. Midline lesions tend to produce truncal and gait ataxia; hemisphere lesions primarily produce limb ataxia.
2. *Cerebellar hemorrhage, infarct, tumor.* There are often occipital headache and ocular gaze palsies. Limb strength and sensa-

tion are preserved. Cerebellar hemorrhage is a neurologic emergency requiring immediate diagnosis (CT scan) and usually surgical intervention (see Chapter 6). Primary cerebellar tumors are seen in childhood; they are rare in adults. Metastatic tumors can involve the cerebellum in adults.

3. Spinocerebellar degeneration. These syndromes include olivopontocerebellar degeneration and Friedreich's ataxia. There is usually a positive family history and evidence of widespread nervous system involvement, e.g., peripheral neuropathy (loss of reflexes), pyramidal tract dysfunction (up-going toes). Pes cavus or scoliosis is sometimes associated with these entities.

4. Alcoholism or occult malignancy may be associated with cerebellar degeneration. Alcoholic cerebellar degeneration is characterized by ataxia of gait and of the legs, with less prominent involvement of arms, speech, or ocular motility. There is usually an associated memory loss and polyneuropathy. Acute ataxia and oculomotor paralysis associated with alcoholism (Wernicke's encephalopathy) respond to thiamine administration (see Chapter 25). Remember, cerebellar ataxia as a "remote" effect may be the presenting symptom of an occult malignancy (see Chapter 21), especially carcinoma of the breast or ovary. Check for anti-Yo antibodies in serum or CSF.

5. Acute cerebellitis is a viral or postviral cause of ataxia sometimes seen in children and rarely in adults.

IS THE LESION IN THE SPINAL CORD ?

(Mechanism: ataxia via posterior column dysfunction, involvement of pyramidal tracts.) Remember, a positive Romberg sign (unsteady with eyes closed, steady with eyes open) usually indicates posterior column disease. MRI is usually diagnostic.

1. Cervical spondylosis with associated cervical myelopathy. Patients usually have neck and arm pain and abnormal cervical spine films. Depending on the extent of spinal cord involvement, there may be posterior column dysfunction and up-going toes (pyramidal tract involvement). MRI is usually diagnostic.

2. Multiple sclerosis often involves the spinal cord. Diagnosis is

made on the basis of finding multiple lesions of the nervous system (e.g., optic neuritis, brainstem signs) and a history of prior attacks. Usually, there is elevation of CSF gamma globulin and abnormal brain MRI. Sometimes in MS, progressive spinal cord dysfunction occurs in the absence of involvement elsewhere in the nervous system.

3. Vitamin B_{12} deficiency may produce combined system disease, i.e., involvement of posterior and lateral columns of the spinal cord. Patients first notice generalized weakness and paresthesias. Later, there is leg stiffness and ataxia. Loss of vibration and position sense occurs, associated with upgoing toes and often, diminished or absent knee and ankle jerks, secondary to peripheral neuropathy. There may be mental changes (see Chapter 10).

4. Syringomyelia is a chronic, progressive disorder of spinal cord and at times, medulla (syringobulbia). Cavitation within the substance of the spinal cord causes sensory dissociation (pain and temperature loss with preservation of touch and position sense), anterior horn cell involvement (muscle wasting and fasciculations, absent reflexes in the upper extremities), corticospinal tract involvement (spasticity), and trophic disorders secondary to involvement of spinal sympathetic fibers. Patients often have scoliosis. Syringomyelia may be congenital or acquired (e.g., post-traumatic). Syringes are now well visualized on MRI.

5. Other causes of ataxia secondary to spinal cord dysfunction include spinal cord tumor, spinocerebellar degeneration, tabes dorsalis, and amyotrophic lateral sclerosis.

IS THE LESION IN PERIPHERAL NERVE ?

(Mechanism: ataxia secondary to weakness and, in idiopathic polyneuritis, due to dorsal root involvement.)

1. Idiopathic polyneuritis (Guillain-Barré). The Guillain-Barré syndrome may present as ataxia in its early stages or, if the polyneuritis is mild, be its major clinical manifestation. Diagnosis is based on absent reflexes, increased CSF protein, and slowed nerve conduction times (see Chapter 15). Ataxia may also be a feature of severe peripheral neuropathies from other causes (sensory ataxia).

IS THE LESION IN *MUSCLE*?

(Mechanism: ataxia secondary to muscle weakness.)

Myopathy, whether acquired (e.g., polymyositis, thyroid myopathy) or congenital (muscular dystrophy), may be associated with ataxia. Diagnosis is made on the basis of physical examination, muscle enzymes, and muscle biopsy (see Chapter 16).

Rarer causes of *chronic progressive ataxia* include Charcot-Marie-Tooth disease, Ramsay Hunt syndrome, familial spastic ataxia and Huntington's chorea. Ataxia may be associated with Refsum's syndrome (a genetic disorder due to a defect in phytanic acid metabolism), abetalipoproteinemia (Bassen-Kornzweig syndrome), juvenile dystonic lipidosis, meningeal leukemia, occult neuroblastoma, and hypothyroidism.

Acute forms have been associated with drug and chemical ingestions (e.g., alcohol, lead), acute labyrinthitis, postictal states, sickle cell crisis, and lupus erythematosus. The rapidity of onset, other clinical features, and laboratory findings usually permit rapid differentiation of acute ataxia from the chronic forms.

In addition to a careful history and physical examination, the CT scan and MRI are invaluable in the *diagnosis* of ataxia secondary to cerebellar infarct or hemorrhage, cerebellar or frontal lobe tumor, and normal pressure hydrocephalus. Other studies, such as CSF gamma globulin in multiple sclerosis, vitamin B_{12} level in pernicious anemia, and cervical spine films for cervical spondylosis, are obtained when these diagnoses are suspected on clinical grounds.

Suggested Readings

Gilman S, Newman S. Manter & Gatz's essentials of clinical neuroanatomy and neurophysiology. 7th ed. Philadelphia: FA Davis, 1987.

Rosenberg RN, Grossman AG. Hereditary ataxia. Neurol Clin 1989;7:25–36.

Chapter 19

Peripheral Nerve and Root Dysfunction

To diagnose peripheral nerve and root injuries, one must determine which muscles are affected and the territory of the sensory loss. Thus, one must know which roots and nerves supply which muscles, and their sensory distribution.

REFLEXES

Reflexes are diminished in root and peripheral nerve disease. (Root irritation alone or damage to a root not involved in the reflex arc does not decrease the reflex.) There are four primary reflexes to remember, with particular roots and muscles necessary for their function. An easy way to learn the roots is to remember that, going from ankle to triceps, the roots are numbered consecutively from one to eight.

ROOTS AND MUSCLES

There is an overlap between roots and the muscles they supply; thus, more than one root is generally responsible for each muscle. Nevertheless, certain muscles serve as standard clinical indices for each root so that if one particular root is out, there should be one muscle (or muscle group) that is particularly weak.

Each root has a sensory distribution as represented on the standard dermatome chart (see Chapter 30).

Table 19.1.
Four Primary Reflexes

Reflex	Roots Needed for Reflex	Muscle Carrying out the Relex
Ankle jerk	S1	Gastrocnemius
Knee jerk	L2, L3, L4	Quadriceps
Biceps	C5, C6	Biceps
Triceps	C7, C8	Triceps

Table 19.2.
Roots and the Primary Muscles They Supply

Root	Muscle	Action
C5	Deltoid	Shoulder abduction
C5	Infraspinatus	Humeral external rotation (Check: Have patient externally rotate the humerus with the arm held at side and flexed at the elbow, as if shooting a gun)
C5, C6	Biceps	Flexion of the supinated forearm
C6	Extensor carpi radialus and ulnaris	Wrist extension
C7	Extensors digitorum Triceps	Finger extensions; forearm extension at elbow
C8, T1	Interossei and lumbricals	Digital abduction and adduction (Check: have patient move fingers apart and together against resistance)
L2, L3, L4	Quadriceps Iliopsoas Adductor group	Knee extension Thigh on hip flexion Thigh adduction
L5	Anterior tibial and extensor hallucis	Ankle and large toe dorsiflexion (Check: have patient walk on heels)
S1	Gastrocnemius	Ankle plantar flexion (Check: have walk on tiptoes)

NERVES AND MUSCLES OF THE UPPER EXTREMITY

Median Nerve

The median nerve (C6-T1) originates in the shoulder (brachial plexus) and supplies two basic muscle groups:

Table 19.3.
Characteristic Features Associated with Various Nerves

Nerve	Involvement
Median	Thumb and thenar eminence
Ulnar	Little finger and hypothenar eminence
Radial	Wrist-drop
Femoral	Absent knee jerk (weak hip flexion and knee extension)
Peroneal	Foot-drop
Sciatic	Pain down lateral thigh and leg, often with absent ankle jerk

- *Forearm:* pronator of the forearm, radial flexion, and wrist abduction.
- *Hand:* first two *L*umbricales (index and middle finger flexion at the metacarpophalangeal joint); thumb *O*pposition with opponens pollicis, *A*bduction with abductor pollicis brevis, and *F*lexion with flexor pollicis brevis ("LOAF" muscles.)

Sensory loss involves the thumb, index, middle, and half of the ring finger.

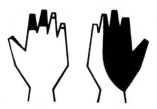

Clinical comment: A complete median nerve lesion (both forearm and hand muscles) is usually secondary to traumatic injury in the axilla or a lesion affecting the median nerve at the elbow. Partial involvement (at the wrist), one of the most frequently encountered mononeuropathies, is termed the *carpal tunnel syndrome* (as median nerve is compressed in carpal tunnel). Patients will often complain of numbness and tingling in the thumb and first two fingers; muscle wasting and loss of power (thenar eminence) occur later. The diagnosis may be confirmed by nerve conduction studies. The carpal tunnel syndrome is often bilateral and may be associated with systemic processes; look for rheumatoid arthritis, myxedema, diabetes, pregnancy, gout, acromegaly, and amyloidosis. Medical management includes treating the underlying disease, administering diuretics, splinting the wrist, and injection of steroids into the carpal tunnel. Surgical decompression of the carpal tunnel may be necessary and is usually successful.

> When median nerve involvement is suspected, think of thumb and thenar eminence.

Ulnar Nerve

The ulnar nerve (C8-T1) is the counterpart of the median nerve in the forearm and hand. It supplies all muscles and sensory areas (on palm) not supplied by the median nerve. When ulnar nerve disease is suspected, think of little finger and hypothenar eminence. The ulnar nerve runs in the ulnar groove at the medial aspect of the elbow ("funny bone") and supplies the following two muscle groups:

- *Forearm:* ulnar flexion at the wrist.
- *Hand:* little finger abduction and opposition, thumb adduction, all the interosseous muscles (used to spread fingers apart and bring together); third and fourth lumbricales (ring and little finger flexion at the metacarpophalangeal joint).

Sensory loss involves the fourth and little finger.

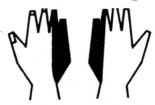

Clinical comment: Ulnar nerve palsy gives a "claw hand" deformity with extension of the ring and little fingers (ability to flex is lost). The ulnar nerve is commonly injured at the elbow, where it is most exposed. Tardive (or delayed) ulnar palsy may occur years after trauma to the elbow (perhaps when fibrosis becomes significant). Look for muscle weakness as opposed to the prominent sensory symptoms seen in median nerve dysfunction. A claw hand is also seen with involvement of C8-T1 roots at the origin of the brachial plexus due to trauma, surgery, or tumor at the apex of the lung. Check for Horner's syndrome (small pupil and ptosis) on the same side as the claw hand. This indicates sympathetic fiber involvement in the area of the brachial plexus.

Radial Nerve

The radial nerve (C5-C8) winds around the lateral aspect of the elbow. When one suspects radial nerve involvement, think of wrist-drop.

The radial nerve supplies these muscles:

- *Supinator* of the forearm. The brachioradialis reflex may be lost.
- *Extensors* of the fingers, wrist, elbow (triceps), and thumb.

Sensory loss involves the back of the hand and is not always present.

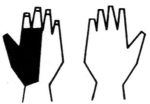

Clinical comment: Injury to the radial nerve may occur in the axilla (e.g., after using crutches) giving inability to extend the elbow plus wrist-drop. If the radial nerve is involved at the elbow, only wrist-drop is found. Pressure palsies are common ("Saturday night palsy" and "bridegroom's palsy," when the groom sleeps with bride's head on his arm). In addition, the radial nerve is affected in diabetes and lead poisoning. In radial nerve palsy, the ability to spread the fingers apart (ulnar nerve function) may be weak due to the mechanical disadvantage caused by the wrist-drop. Check with wrist resting on a flat surface (e.g., table) to overcome that handicap.

Cervical discs

Herniated discs causing nerve root compression are less common in the cervical than in the lumbar area. They should be suspected when a patient's sensory findings and/or symptoms conform to a particular root distribution and are accompanied by reflex and motor dysfunction of the same root. Note associated neck pain.

Cervical Spondylosis

Check for (a) multiple, often asymmetrical root involvement in the upper extremities, with muscle wasting and hypoactive reflexes in the distribution of those roots affected; (b) compression of the cervical spinal cord, giving hyperactive lower extremity reflexes, up-going toes, and later, leg weakness. Remember, sensory symptoms in the hands plus spastic lower extremities in patients over 50 equal cervical spondylosis with myelopathy until proven otherwise (check vitamin B_{12} level). Similar symptoms may be caused by foramen magnum tumors or anomalies of the posterior fossa such as Chiari malformations, especially in younger patients.

NERVES AND MUSCLES OF THE LOWER EXTREMITY

The obturator nerve (L2-L3-L4 roots, ventral portion) supplies the adductors of the thigh. It may be damaged during labor, involved in diabetes, or affected by local pelvic disease or by obturator hernia.

Femoral Nerve

The femoral nerve (L2-L3-L4 roots, dorsal portion) supplies the iliopsoas (hip flexion) and quadriceps (knee extension). The knee jerk is diminished or absent. Femoral nerve involvement may be distinguished from root involvement at L2-L3-L4 (e.g., by paravertebral tumor) by checking thigh adduction (obturator), which is affected if roots are involved but spared if the femoral nerve alone is involved. Causes of femoral neuropathy include diabetes (look for quadriceps wasting with pain over the anterior, "diabetic amyotrophy" thigh), tumor, polyarteritis, pelvic trauma, and hemorrhage into the iliacus muscle in patients on anticoagulants.

Lateral Femoral Cutaneous Nerve

This pure sensory nerve (L2-L3) supplies the lateral thigh. There is tingling, burning, and pain. The lateral femoral cutaneous nerve syndrome (meralgia paraesthetica) is common in diabetes, and may appear during pregnancy or as a result of pressure from a corset, a tight-fitting belt, obesity, or even poor posture. Treatment involves removing the offending agent, and, if necessary, injection of the nerve at its entrance to the thigh with lidocaine (Xylocaine) and steroids, or surgical transection.

Sciatic Nerve

The sciatic nerve (L4-S3) supplies hamstrings (flexion of the knee) and all muscles below the knee.

At the knee it divides into the:

Peroneal, which runs anteriorly and supplies muscles that dorsiflex and evert the foot and sensation on top of the foot.

Posterior tibial, which runs posteriorly at the knee and supplies muscles of plantar flexion and inversion and sensation on the sole of the foot.

Clinically, the most common affliction of the sciatic nerve is sciatica, a painful sensory disturbance beginning in the buttock and moving down the lateral aspect of the thigh. Irritation of any root from L4-S3 may produce sciatica to a varying degree. One of the most common causes of sciatica is lumbar disc protrusion (pain may be precipitated by coughing or sneezing), often with associated reflex loss and weakness in a root distribution. Straight leg raising generally aggravates the back pain. Some patients may have no neurologic findings with a herniated disc, although often there is paravertebral muscle spasm.

The decision to carry out myelography, CT scan, MRI, and/or surgery for lumbar disc disease depends on the ability to relieve pain with bed rest (10–14 days of complete bed rest are usually necessary) and physical therapy and the presence of weakness or other abnormal neurológic signs. Some have advocated short courses of high-dose dexamethasone for disc disease.

Table 19.4.
Most Common Lumbar Disc Syndromes

Root	Disc Interspace	Reflex Affected	Motor Weakness	Sensory Changes (if any)
L4	L3–L4	Knee jerk	Knee extension	Anterior thigh
L5	L4–L5	Hamstring jerk	Large toe dorsiflexion	Large toe
S1	L5–S1	Ankle jerk	Foot, plantar flexion	Foot, lateral border

Peroneal Nerve

The peroneal nerve supplies dorsiflexors (tibialis anterior) and everters (turning out) of the foot. (Inverters (turning in) of the foot are supplied by the posterior tibial nerve.) The sensory distribution involves the lateral aspect of the leg and dorsum of the foot.

Clinically, peroneal nerve palsy gives foot-drop and is analogous to wrist-drop (radial nerve) in the upper extremity. Foot-drop is seen in diabetes and is a frequent pressure palsy from either trauma or pressure in a thin or wasted individual (because of the superficial location of the nerve at the lateral aspect of the knee). Hereditary peroneal neuropathy (Charcot-Marie-Tooth disease) is associated with bilateral foot-drop, a wasted anterior leg compartment below the knee, and pes cavus. Remember, peroneal palsy spares the inverters of the foot; if they too are weak, the lesion is higher, generally at the root, sciatic nerve, or cord level. Though peroneal palsy is the most common cause of foot-drop, the *differential diagnosis of foot-drop includes:*

1. Sciatic nerve injury—*Clue:* Tibialis posterior affected as are other muscles, such as gastrocnemius, supplied by sciatic nerve.
2. L5 nerve root—*Clue:* Tibialis posterior affected, often with associated back pain.
3. Spinal cord—*Clue:* Upper motor neuron signs (e.g. Babinski) present.

4. Hemisphere—Clue: Anterior cerebral infarct causes other signs of hemiparesis and frontal lobe signs.

An EMG and nerve conduction study are useful in establishing the diagnosis and prognosis in foot-drop.

Posterior Tibial Nerve

This nerve is rarely injured alone, because it runs deep in the calf. It may be entrapped distally in the tarsal tunnel, causing pain in the sole of the foot.

Table 19.5.

	Conus medullaris	Cauda equina
Motor weakness	Absent or mild	Present and usually unilateral
Sensory deficits	Bilateral (saddle)	Usually unilateral
Sphincter involvement	Early; of bladder and bowel	Late and mild
Differential diagnosis	Tumor, hemmorrhage disc, pelvic fracture spondylolisthesis	Same

CONUS MEDULLARIS AND CAUDA EQUINA LESIONS

The conus medullaris (lower sacral segments of the spinal cord) and cauda equina (elongated roots of the lumbar and sacral spinal nerves) can each be affected by a variety of processes. Helpful distinguishing features are contained in Table 19.5.

INVESTIGATION OF NERVE AND ROOT DYSFUNCTION

Examine the patient to determine whether the nerve or root is involved. Determine whether the sensory loss (or symptom) and muscle weakness (if present) fit the distribution of a particular nerve or root.

Establish the *etiology*. If a particular nerve or root is definitely involved, determine the specific etiologic factors unique to that nerve or root. The following questions are important to ask:

1. Did a nerve palsy come on after *sleep* or *surgery* (pressure palsies)?
2. Is there evidence of *trauma*, old or new?
3. What are the patient's *occupation* and habits? For example, there may be median nerve involvement in gardeners and beauty operators or ulnar nerve damage in cornhuskers.
4. Is there evidence of *systemic disease* (e.g., diabetes, uremia, breast cancer affecting the brachial plexus, polyarteritis, granulomatous infection, human immunodeficiency virus infection, nutritional deficiency).

TRIGEMINAL NEURALGIA (Tic Douloureux)

Excruciating, paroxysmal pain lasting seconds to minutes in the distribution of the second or third division of the fifth cranial nerve is the hallmark of trigeminal neuralgia. The pain is often "triggered" by touching the side of the face or brought on by facial movement, such as chewing. There is no objective motor or sensory loss. The cause is unknown but may be related to a viral infection or to pressure on the nerve by a basilar artery branch near the brainstem. Trigeminal neuralgia is uncommon in people under 40. When it occurs in the younger patient, particularly if associated with objective sensory loss, it is frequently secondary to multiple sclerosis. Neurologic signs (loss of sensation on the face, cranial nerve palsies, long tract signs) suggest focal pathology, such as tumor, vascular malformation, or demyelinating disease. Treatment with carbamazepine (Tegretol) relieves pain in most patients (begin with 100 mg twice a day; increase by 100 mg/day up to 1200 mg/day; monitor hematologic indices). Other drugs, such as phenytoin or baclofen may also be useful. Patients refractory to medical treatment require surgical intervention. Percutaneous radiofrequency coagulation of the gasserian ganglion may be extremely effective in relieving the pain of trigeminal neuralgia, and some patients have had vascular decompression of the trigeminal nerve via craniotomy.

SEVENTH NERVE PALSIES, INCLUDING BELL'S PALSY

Peripheral involvement of the seventh cranial nerve is a well-recognized syndrome. Onset may be heralded by pain behind the ear, and diagnosis is based on demonstrating complete facial palsy, i.e., paralysis of both lower face and forehead, in the absence of other neurologic findings. Central lesions that affect fibers prior to their synapse in the seventh nerve nucleus in the brainstem spare forehead musculature. In addition to innervating facial musculature, fibers from the seventh nerve innervate the lacrimal gland of the eye (decreasing tearing), the stapedius muscle in the ear (hyperacusis), the submaxillary and sublingual glands and carry afferent taste fibers from the anterior two-thirds of the tongue (loss of taste). Most cases are idiopathic (Bell's palsy). Other causes include infectious mononucleosis, Lyme disease, the Guillain-Barré syndrome (bilateral seventh nerve palsies, loss of reflexes), fracture, severe hypertension, diabetes, sarcoid and histiocytosis, and an associated otitis or mastoiditis. A cerebellopontine angle tumor or a brainstem plaque from multiple sclerosis may give a peripheral seventh nerve palsy, usually in association with other cranial nerve signs. Melkersson's syndrome is recurrent seventh nerve palsies associated with facial edema.

Treatment with prednisone probably hastens recovery and the amount of residual facial disfiguration in the idiopathic (Bell's palsy) variety and should be given within the first 72 hours of onset: 60 mg daily for 4 days, then taper to 5 mg/day in 10 days. Eye patching and methylcellulose eye drops will help prevent corneal ulceration. Surgical decompression probably is of no benefit. Recovery usually begins within 1 to 4 weeks of onset and may take longer than 3 months to be complete. Patients with hyperacusis, taste loss, or defective tearing have a poorer prognosis (proximal lesion of the facial nerve) as do those with complete (as opposed to partial) facial nerve paralysis. Remember to perform a careful neurologic examination in search of other neurologic signs in patients with a peripheral seventh nerve palsy.

THORACIC OUTLET SYNDROME

The *thoracic outlet syndrome* refers to symptoms and signs that occur due to compression of the subclavian vessels and brachial plexus at the superior aperture of the thorax between the first rib and the clavicle. Symptoms include pain and paresthesias in the neck, shoulder, arm, and hand (C8, T1 distribution), weakness of the hand, change of color of the hand, including pallor of the fingers, and aggravation of all symptoms by use of the upper limb. Signs depend on whether primarily vascular or neural compression exists and include supraclavicular bruit, loss or diminution of radial pulse, weakness and sensory loss in the hand, and reproduction of pain by pressure in the supraclavicular fossa or by traction on the arm. Anomalies of the spine are often present, including cervical ribs or abnormal transverse process of C7.

Suggested Readings

Adour KK. Diagnosis and management of facial paralysis. N Engl J Med 1982;307:348.

Aids to the investigation of peripheral nerve injuries. London: Her Majesty's Stationery Office, 1986.

Dawson DM. Entrapment neuropathies. Boston: Little, Brown & Co, 1990.

Dyck PJ. The causes, classification and treatment of peripheral neuropathy. N Engl J Med 1982;307:283.

Fromm JH. Trigeminal neuralgia and related disorders. Neurol Clin 1989;7(2):305–320.

Sunderland S. Nerves and nerve injuries. London: Churchill Livingstone, 1978.

Chapter 20

Neurology of Diabetes

Diabetes frequently manifests a variety of neurologic symptoms; indeed, "neuropathy" is a classic diabetic complication. Most of the neurologic complications of diabetes are not referable to the central nervous system. Cerebrovascular disease, although more common in diabetes, is not a diabetic phenomenon—but one to which the diabetic is prone.

DIABETIC "NEUROPATHY"

Polyneuropathy

Polyneuropathy is the most common diabetic neuropathy; it manifests as a symmetrical, distal ("glove and stocking") sensory polyneuropathy, sparing motor function. The upper border of the sensory loss is irregular; ankle jerks are generally absent, and vibration sense is diminished. This benign neuropathy usually does not bring the patient to the physician and, apart from minor paresthesias, is asymptomatic. It can, however, lead to trophic changes and injury from trauma, infection, ulceration, and rarely joint destruction, because of the loss of pain sensation. Rarely, it is painful.

Mononeuropathy

Mononeuropathy is a dramatic diabetic neuropathy that probably results from nerve infarction. The onset of motor and sensory loss in one nerve is abrupt and often painful; the involved nerve may be tender. Prognosis is good, and recovery usually occurs in 4–6 months. Treatment is with physical therapy and appropriate support (splints where needed).

There is a predilection for certain nerves. The most commonly affected are:

1. Oculomotor (III) nerve. The patient has diplopia and may have pain over the eye. There is an almost total ophthalmoplegia (lateral eye movement is spared). The clue to a "diabetic third" is that the pupillary fibers are usually spared. (The pupillary fibers are on the outer perimeter of the nerve, and vascular infarction occurs centrally.) Thus, the pupil is of normal size and reacts. It is not large and unreactive as in other third nerve palsies (e.g., those due to compression).

2. Abducens (VI) nerve. There is an isolated inability to move the eye laterally. Remember, a sixth nerve palsy may also be the first sign of increased intracranial pressure (check for headache and papilledema).

3. Femoral nerve. There is pain in the lateral and anterior thigh; weakness and atrophy of quadriceps (extension at knee) plus weakness of iliopsoas (flexion of hip); and a diminished or absent knee jerk (see Chapter 19).

4. Radial nerve and peroneal nerve. There is wrist-drop or foot-drop (see Chapter 19).

5. *Facial (VII) nerve.* Bell's palsy is more common in diabetics (see Chapter 19).

Radiculopathy

Radiculopathy is secondary to involvement of the posterior root outside the spinal cord before it becomes a mixed nerve. Clinically, the patient complains of shooting pains, often confined to one dermatome. There are usually no motor or reflex changes. This neuropathy may be difficult to distinguish from disc disease and fortunately resolves spontaneously. Lumbar and thoracic roots are most frequently affected, and involvement may be bilateral. Sometimes there is posterior column degeneration, resulting in posterior column dysfunction and shooting pains. If the patient has these symptoms plus an irregular pupil that accommodates but reacts poorly to light (sometimes seen in diabetics), the term "diabetic pseudotabes" is used.

Lumbar Plexopathy

Lumbar plexopathy (previously called "amyotrophy") is generally seen in older patients and consists of pain in the thighs and proximal muscle weakness and wasting. Quadriceps and hamstrings may also be weak, and the patient complains of myalgia and dysesthesias in the thighs, although there is usually no objective sensory loss. Knee and ankle reflexes are usually absent. There is evidence to indicate a microvascular ischemic process, with proximal motor nerves of the lower extremities being affected preferentially. The prognosis is good, with recovery occurring over 6–12 months, particularly with optimum control of the diabetes. (Check for other causes of proximal muscle weakness—e.g., endocrine myopathy, polymyositis.)

Autonomic Neuropathy

The most common manifestations of *autonomic neuropathy* are orthostatic hypotension (treat with elastic stockings, mineralocorticoids), nocturnal diarrhea, impotence, urinary retention, and abdominal distension.

COMMENTS ON DIABETES AND THE NERVOUS SYSTEM

There is no specific treatment for the various *diabetic neuropathies*. The physician should make sure that the neuropathies are associated with diabetes and do not represent symptoms due to other treatable processes. Support and physical therapy are important during the period of recovery. There is evidence that neuropathies may be ameliorated by careful blood sugar control in the diabetic and that insulin is more effective than oral agents. Drugs such as amytriptyline, phenytoin, or nonsteroidal antiinflammatory agents may be useful for the pain or paresthesias of diabetic neuropathy. Axain, a topical ointment made from an extract of chili peppers, is effective but quite costly. Experimental trials of drugs involved in the sorbitol pathway, such as inositol, are being performed. Other helpful measures include frequently examining the feet for ulcers or infection; wearing comfortable, well-fitted shoes; and avoiding other toxins such as alcohol to prevent additive neuropathies. Workup of suspected diabetic neuropathy should include assessing duration and control of diabetes and checking for foot deformities and skin changes. Electromyogram and nerve conduction studies are often helpful in differential diagnosis.

CSF protein is frequently elevated in diabetes.

Remember, *spinal fluid protein* is frequently elevated in diabetes.

Diabetic coma and *hypoglycemia* are not discussed in detail here. Remember to draw a blood sugar and administer 50% glucose intravenously to all patients presenting with coma of uncertain cause. Patients with hypoglycemia may present with behavioral disturbances, seizures, and even focal neurologic deficits that clear after glucose administration. Treatment of *hyperglycemia* and coma may result in hypokalemia and a flaccid paralysis.

Diabetics are at increased risk for cerebrovascular disease.

Cervical spondylosis is more apt to be symptomatic in the diabetic than the nondiabetic. There may be hyperactive reflexes at the knees with up-going toes (secondary to compression of the cord at the cervical region), and loss of ankle jerks and vibration sense (secondary to the diabetic neuropathy).

NOTE: Recent studies suggest that certain alcohol sugars are increased in diabetic neuropathy and that aldose reductase inhibitors such as sorbinil, tolrestat, and statil may be of clinical benefit and are worthy of large-scale study.

Suggested Readings

Asbury AK. Understanding diabetic neuropathy. N Engl J Med 1988;319:577.

Cohen J, Gross K. Autonomic neuropathy: clinical presentation and differential diagnosis. Geriatrics 1990;45:33–42.

Greene DA. Diabetic neuropathy. Annu Rev Med 1990;41:303–317.

Harati Y. Diabetic peripheral neuropathies. Ann Intern Med 1987;107:546.

Pirart J. Diabetes mellitus and its degenerative complications. Diabetes Care 1978;1:252–263.

Riddle MC. Diabetic neuropathies in the elderly: management update. Geriatrics 1990;45:32–36.

Chapter 21

Malignancy and the Nervous System

Malignancy may affect the nervous system in two ways: (*a*) by direct involvement of either primary or metastatic brain or spinal cord tumor; and (*b*) by nonmetastatic effects, when nervous system dysfunction is associated with malignancy elsewhere in the body. The prevalence of neurologic complications of cancer is increasing with improvement of treatment and increased longevity in patients with cancer.

SIGNS AND SYMPTOMS OF BRAIN TUMOR

These signs and symptoms apply to both primary and metastatic CNS tumors.

1. Does the patient have *headache?* This is one of the most common symptoms, being present in about two-thirds of patients. It often occurs in the morning, when intracranial pressure is higher.
2. Other signs and symptoms include seizures, personality changes, hemiplegia, and visual disturbances. Mental changes, especially memory loss and decreased alertness are often important subtle clues of intracranial tumor.
3. Patients may have a *gait disturbance.*
4. *Seizures* associated with tumor are characteristically focal. They may be jacksonian: a focal seizure that begins in one extremity and then "marches" until it becomes a generalized convulsion.

5. Check for *papilledema* or sixth nerve paresis due to raised intracranial pressure.
6. Sometimes there may be bleeding within a tumor or vessel occlusion, creating the clinical picture of a stroke. Some tumors have a propensity to bleed (e.g., melanoma, hypernephroma, choriocarcinoma).

INTRACRANIAL METASTASES

Which Tumors Invade the Brain?

Metastatic tumor reaches the brain via hematogenous spread and generally after first invading the lung. This accounts for the high incidence of intracranial metastases with *lung* and *breast* tumors. Tumors of the gastrointestinal tract may metastasize to the brain, although they do so less frequently and generally invade the liver and lung first. *Hypernephroma* and *melanoma* are important sources of CNS metastases but are less common tumors. *Prostatic* carcinoma, a common tumor in elderly men, rarely goes to the brain.

> Prostatic cancer rarely metastasizes to the brain.

Theoretically, metastases might occur via Batson's venous plexus near the lower spinal cord, but the rarity of prostatic metastases to brain demonstrates how nonfunctional this route actually is. Tumors of the *cervix* and *ovary* also metastasize to the brain infrequently.

When Do Tumors Metastasize to the Brain?

Most metastases occur within 2 years of discovery of the primary lesion, although they can sometimes appear years after the removal of a primary source (e.g., with kidney or breast cancer). Conversely, a metastatic tumor may be the first sign of a primary neoplasm elsewhere, especially with lung cancer.

When a neurologic symptom (e.g., seizure) is secondary to a brain metastasis, obvious neurologic progression will usually occur within 6 months. For example, a patient with known breast carcinoma who has a convulsion and then remains neurologically intact for 6 months probably did not experience the seizure because of a cerebral metastasis.

LABORATORY INVESTIGATION

1. MRI with gadolinium enhancement is the most sensitive test for detection of brain tumor especially in the posterior fossa. Contrast-enhanced CT is also very accurate. Contrast-enhanced MRI is particularly useful if leptomeningeal metastases are suspected. An EEG is often abnormal and shows focal slowing with hemisphere tumor. An LP should not be performed if an intracranial tumor is suspected (see Chapter 29).

2. Arteriography is rarely necessary for diagnosis, though it may help in distinguishing primary from metastatic lesions. There is increasing use of stereotactic brain biopsy as a method of establishing the correct diagnosis with low morbidity, particularly for lesions that are not considered resectable.

3. The physician must evaluate each patient individually in terms of which studies to perform.

TREATMENT

The treatment of *primary brain tumor* depends on the tumor type and location. Meningiomas are usually removable. Low-grade astrocytomas and oligodendrogliomas are best treated by surgery plus irradiation. High-grade astrocytomas (glioblastoma multiforme) are treated by resection plus irradiation or, depending on location, partial removal plus irradiation. There is increasing use of chemotherapy (e.g., BCNU), which prolongs survival.

In the approach to patients with *metastatic brain tumor*, one must first determine whether the brain is involved by single or multiple metastases. Documented *multiple metastases* are treated with steroids and whole brain irradiation. Symptoms are ameliorated with steroids (to reduce cerebral edema). Irradiation improves both length and quality of survival. Chemotherapy may be added. Treatment of a *single metastasis* is controversial. Some authors advocate surgical removal; in addition to offering palliation, other processes are sometimes found at operation (e.g., subdural hematoma, abscess, primary brain tumor). Nevertheless, the associated risks of craniotomy are real, and often there are multiple metastases that were not revealed by laboratory investigation. MRI now allows more precise diagnosis of multiple metastases, making this decision easier.

The choice of treatment (surgery, steroids, or irradiation) for the patient with a single metastasis depends on the extent and nature of the primary tumor, the patient's individual circumstances (e.g., age and medical condition), and the philosophy of the primary physician and neurologist or neurosurgeon.

METASTATIC TUMOR TO THE SPINAL CORD

Management

Metastatic tumor to the cord (generally epidural implant) may compress the cord; it constitutes a neurologic emergency. Carcinoma of the lung, breast, or prostate or lymphomas and leukemias may cause spinal cord compression. Back pain, tenderness, change in urinary frequency, or symptoms or root involvement often appear prior to compression. Plain films of the spine usually are abnormal, but the findings may be subtle. Thus, MRI or bone scan is often helpful. See Chapter 14 for evaluation and treatment of acute spinal cord compression.

LEUKEMIA AND LYMPHOMA

These malignant processes are frequently associated with nervous system dysfunction and may invade the brain and spinal cord. With more effective treatment and with patients living longer, there has been an increasing incidence of CNS complications.

Leukemia

Leukemia is associated with a triad of neurologic complications.

1. *Intracranial hemorrhage* is common in leukemia (often fatal) and is usually related to a low platelet count or a high leukocyte count (above 100,000/mm). Intracranial bleeding occurs in multiple areas (not usually one, as in hypertensive bleeding) and is often associated with systemic bleeding. Once bleeding has occurred, transfusion therapy is of little benefit. Therefore, it is crucial to maintain hematologic

indices as normal as possible before neurologic complications occur.

2. *Leukemic infiltration* of meninges (both of brain and spinal cord) and nerve roots is common and frequently occurs when the patient is in hematologic remission. Meningeal leukemia usually presents as headache, nausea, and vomiting secondary to raised intracranial pressure (there may be papilledema); seizures, visual disturbances, and ataxia also occur. Cranial nerve palsies occur and commonly involve the oculomotor (III), abducens (VI), and facial (VII) nerves. *Diagnosis* is made by lumbar puncture. Check for leukemic cells, elevated protein, decreased sugar, and an elevated pressure. Contrast-enhanced MRI may detect leukemic infiltration and is particularly useful in detecting leptomeningeal spread. Treatment with intrathecal methotrexate and radiotherapy is usually effective and may be given prophylactically to leukemic patients in hematologic remission, before CNS complications occur.

NOTE: The hypothalamic-pituitary axis may be involved, resulting in hyperphagia (weight gain) or diabetes insipidus. In addition, there may be infiltration surrounding cord and roots; look for signs and symptoms of cord compression and/or root dysfunction.

3. *Infection.* These patients are prone to CNS infection—bacterial (*Listeria*) and fungal (*Cryptococcus*). Whenever CNS symptoms are present, even if only drowsiness and headache, perform an LP to look for meningeal leukemia or infection, after excluding a mass lesion by CT scan or MRI.

NOTE: Herpes zoster is common, at times affecting roots with prior leukemic infiltration.

Lymphoma

Patients with *lymphoma* are subject to the same complications as those with leukemia, except for intracerebral hemorrhage.

Spinal cord compression by lymphoma is especially common, as are compressive syndromes in other parts of the nervous system: brachial plexus, recurrent laryngeal nerve (vocal cord paralysis), phrenic nerve, cervical sympathetics (Horner's syndrome), and lumbosacral roots. Treatment of choice is radiation. The compressive syndromes are more common in lymphomas than in leukemias.

Although intracerebral lymphoma is rare, it has been reported with reticulum cell sarcoma (histiocytic lymphoma).

Primary central nervous system lymphoma is frequently encountered in AIDS patients. In these patients, differentiation of lymphoma from toxoplasmosis is a common problem (see Chapter 23). In some instances stereotactic biopsy may be needed.

NOTE: Meningeal involvement by tumors other than lymphoma and leukemia (*carcinomatous meningitis*) occurs most commonly with breast cancer. As with meningeal leukemia (see above), look for symptoms of raised intracranial pressure, multiple cranial nerve palsies, radiculopathy, and cerebrospinal fluid abnormalities (malignant cells and high protein). Treatment consists of intrathecal chemotherapy and radiotherapy. Placing an Ommaya reservoir for injecting the drug(s) is often recommended.

NONMETASTATIC COMPLICATIONS OF MALIGNANCY

"Remote" effects. This unique group of symptoms reflects the remote effects of malignancy on the nervous system. The etiology of these distant effects varies and may be related to immunologic, hormonal, or toxic factors elaborated by the tumor.

> Neurologic syndromes may be the first manifestation of a malignancy elsewhere.

It is known, however, that these neurologic syndromes may be the first manifestation of a malignancy elsewhere (e.g., peripheral neuropathy associated with lung tumor), and they sometimes disappear when the primary tumor is removed. Certain neoplasms are more commonly associated with neurologic findings. However, as more syndromes are being reported, a wider spectrum of "etiologic malignancies" is becoming apparent.

Cerebellar Degeneration

Clinically, there is unsteadiness in gait and difficulty using limbs, progressing to slurred speech and trouble eating. Nystagmus may not be present. Cerebellar degeneration has been reported with tumors of lung, ovary, breast, and colon and with lymphoma. Although the cerebellar dysfunction is most striking, there may be other evidence of associated CNS dysfunction, including mental changes, muscle weakness, and extensor plantar responses. Anti–Purkinje cell antibodies have been detected in the serum and CSF of these patients.

Myasthenic (Eaton-Lambert) Syndrome

This syndrome is most frequently associated with small cell lung tumor in men. It presents as generalized weakness and easy fatigability, the weakness being most prominent proximally. Associated features include dry mouth, impotence, and peripheral paresthesias. Trouble with eye movements or difficulty swallowing is less common. The characteristic feature of this syndrome is that a few muscle contractions must be carried out before full strength is reached, after which the patient fatigues. (In myasthenia gravis, full strength is present at the outset and diminishes with exercise.) This can be demonstrated by electrodiagnostic studies. Eaton-Lambert is a presynaptic disorder of the neuromuscular junction; myasthenia gravis affects the postsynaptic junction. Treatment with guanidine (which facilitates acetylcholine release) is more beneficial than anticholinesterase medication. The myasthenic syndrome may occur in the absence of malignancy; evidence suggests an autoimmune basis for this syndrome.

Sensory Neuropathy

There is numbness and tingling of the upper and lower extremities associated with a sensory ataxia. Reflexes are absent, and there may be proximal muscle wasting in the lower extremities. A sensorimotor neuropathy has also been associated with malignancy.

Opsoclonus-Myoclonus

Opsoclonus, a peculiar jerking of the eyes to and fro, and myoclonus, a sudden jerking of large muscle group, may be seen as remote effects of cancer (neuroblastoma).

Dementia

Dementia may be associated with malignancy (carcinoma of the lung), secondary to "limbic encephalitis" which causes severely impaired memory. There may be associated diffuse changes in the nervous system and a concomitant sensory neuropathy.

Polymyositis and Dermatomyositis

Both of these conditions are associated with neoplasm and may antedate the appearance of the tumor. Myositis presents as proximal muscle weakness. The muscles are not usually tender, only weak. If tumor eradication is not possible or does not help, steroids may be of benefit.

Remember, the importance of these remote effects of malignancy is the clue they offer that a malignancy is present, even though they may appear when the tumor is well established. A characteristic feature of these syndromes is that they are seldom "pure"; they spill over to involve more than one area of the nervous system.

Metabolic Encephalopathy

Patients with cancer are prone to develop lethargy, confusion, and behavior disturbances as the result of metabolic abnormalities related to, but not directly resulting from, the underlying cancer. Examples include uremia; hepatic and respiratory failure; electrolyte disturbances, such as hypercalcemia, hyponatremia, hypoglycemia; and drug overdoses. Also, as discussed under "Leukemia," patients with cancer are prone to develop infections of various types, and sepsis may cause a metabolic encephalopathy. Metabolic brain disease is suggested by lethargy, clouding of consciousness, a fluctuating picture, myoclonus, a lack of focal signs, and confirmatory laboratory studies, such as a normal CT scan or MRI and an abnormal EEG that shows bilateral slowing without focal features.

Vascular Disorders

Cancer patients are prone to develop vascular disorders, such as cerebral infarction secondary to disseminated intravascular coagulation, and hypercoagulable states, venous sinus thromboses, or emboli from nonbacterial endocarditis. They are also prone to intracerebral, subarachnoid, or subdural hemorrhage, as discussed under "Leukemia."

Other

Cancer patients may develop side effects of therapy, such as radiation myelopathy, neuropathy, encephalopathy, and peripheral neuropathy secondary to chemotherapeutic agents (especially vincristine and cisplatinum).

NOTE: *Progressive multifocal leukoencephalopathy (PML)* is usually seen in patients with a compromised immune system. This occurs in patients with malignancies such as lymphomas or secondary to immunosuppression from chemotherapy or in AIDS patients. Clinically, patients develop deterioration of mental states, multiple focal neurologic deficits with multifocal white matter lesions over a period of 6 months to 2 years. The clinical picture may be confused with multiple strokes. It is caused by a papovavirus.

Suggested Readings

Anderson NE. Autoantibodies in paraneoplastic syndromes associated with small cell lung cancer. Neurology 1988;38:1391.

Patchell RA, ed. Neurological complications of systemic cancer. Neurologic Clinics. Philadelphia: WB Saunders, 1991;9.

Vick NA, Bigner DD. Neurooncology. Neurol Clin 1985;3.

Woodman R. Primary non-Hodgkin's lymphoma of the brain. Medicine 1985;64:425.

Chapter 22

Central Nervous System Infections

Central nervous system (CNS) infections are suggested by a constellation of symptoms, signs, and laboratory studies. It is beyond the scope of this manual to discuss each CNS infection type individually. Rather, this chapter aims to alert the house officer to consider CNS infection as a diagnostic possibility when certain clinical features coexist, to pursue a definitive diagnosis, and to institute treatment.

HISTORY

The diagnosis of meningitis (inflammation of the meninges) is suggested when history includes:

- Fever
- Headache
- Stiff neck

The diagnosis of encephalitis (evidence of brain parenchymal involvement) is suggested when the history includes:

- Mental status changes (confusion to coma)
- Seizures
- Focal neurologic signs such as paralysis

Often these symptoms coexist in "meningoencephalitis." Pursue the following points in the history:

1. Has there been a recent upper respiratory infection or pneumonia?
2. Has the patient had a recent infectious illness that may progress to meningitis (e.g., otitis media leading to pneumococcal meningitis)?
3. Has the patient been exposed to others with infectious illness (e.g., meningococcus or *Haemophilus influenzae*)?
4. Has there been recent travel to another state (e.g., exposure to mosquitoes causing arbovirus encephalitis) or another country (cysticercosis in Central America)?
5. Was there a prodromal febrile illness (e.g., a preceding febrile illness in herpes simplex encephalitis)?
6. Has there been a subtle personality change and low-grade fever (e.g., in chronic meningitis such as *Cryptococcus*)?
7. What is patient's occupation (e.g., painter exposed to *Cryptococcus* in pigeon droppings)?
8. Does an *underlying disease* predispose the patient to CNS infection?
   - Lymphoma, leukemia
   - Other malignancy
   - Renal failure
   - AIDS and other immunodeficiency states
   - Alcoholism
   - Diabetes
9. Is patient receiving a drug(s) that predisposes to infection?
   - Chemotherapy
   - Immunosuppressant
   - Steroids
10. Has the patient had a recent illness such as mumps or chickenpox that may be followed by meningitis or meningoencephalitis?
11. Has there been a recent head injury (precedes 10% of pneumococcal meningitis)?
12. Has there been a recent neurosurgical procedure or penetrating skull trauma?
13. Has there been a recent insect bite leading to Lyme disease or rickettsial infection, which mimics bacterial meningitis?
14. Does the patient have a history of a positive PPD?

PHYSICAL AND NEUROLOGIC EXAMINATION

1. Check vital signs. Temperature is higher in bacterial than viral CNS infection and may be below normal (tuberculosis). Herpes simplex encephalitis often can result in a high fever (104–105°F) initially. Tachycardia is seen in bacterial and viral CNS infection.

2. Check eardrums and for tenderness over the sinuses.

3. Check for stiff neck. Look for Kernig's sign (with thigh flexed on abdomen patient resists knee extension) or Brudzinski's sign (attempt to flex the neck results in reflex flexion of the knee and hip). Remember that the elderly and infants may have meningitis without prominent meningeal signs.

4. Look for stigmata of chronic liver disease and chronic lung disease as a substrate for CNS infection.

5. Look for peripheral signs of embolization in a patient suspected of having subacute bacterial endocarditis with a mycotic aneurysm.

6. Examine the heart carefully—e.g., changing murmur in subacute bacterial endocarditis with valvular disease as source of septic embolism.

7. Examine for lymph node enlargement or splenomegaly. These signs suggest a lymphoproliferative disorder, in which CNS infections are commonly seen.

8. Is there evidence of CSF rhinorrhea due to a defect or fracture in the cribriform plate? (Check an unexplained nasal discharge for presence of CSF glucose).

9. Examine for petechial or purpuric lesions (e.g., due to meningococcemia).

LABORATORY

1. All meningitis suspects should have a spinal tap as soon as possible. Record the opening pressure. If focal neurologic symptoms or signs are present and brain abscess is a consideration, obtain a contrast-enhanced CT or MRI scan first, but do not allow significant delay when there is a high likelihood of meningitis. See Chapter 29 for a discussion of cerebrospinal fluid examination. In addition, note the following points regarding meningitis and encephalitis.

a. Cerebrospinal fluid pressure is usually moderately elevated in bacterial meningitis (200–300 mm H_2O) and mildly elevated in viral meningitis or encephalitis.

b. Cell count in untreated bacterial meningitis is 100–10,000/mm³ with a predominance of polys, and the fluid is usually cloudy. In viral meningitis, cell counts of 10–1,000/mm³ with a predominance of mononuclear cells are expected.

c. CSF glucose is usually below 40 mg/100 ml in bacterial or tuberculous meningitis (less than 60% of simultaneously obtained blood glucose), whereas it is usually *normal* or modestly reduced in viral meningitis or encephalitis.

d. CSF protein is usually elevated above 100 mg/100 ml in bacterial meningitis, whereas a mild elevation (50–100 mg/100 ml) is expected in viral meningitis or encephalitis. A mild elevation may also be seen in a partially treated meningitis.

e. Gram stain usually detects the organism in bacterial meningitis. India ink stain is helpful in cryptococcal meningitis. Bacterial antigens can now be detected in the spinal fluid by a variety of special techniques, which are particularly helpful if the patient received antibiotic therapy prior to the LP.

2. Routine laboratory tests may offer clues. White blood cell count is markedly elevated in bacterial meningitis and mildly elevated in viral meningitis.

3. Check for hyponatremia due to inappropriate ADH secretion as a complicating feature in a patient with meningitis with increasing lethargy.

4. Chest x-ray may demonstrate a source of CNS infection—e.g., due to bronchiectasis.

5. The electroencephalogram is usually normal or slightly slow in meningitis and encephalitis, but it often shows focal features in brain abscess, and paroxysmal features in the temporal lobe in herpes simplex encephalitis.

6. CT scan is usually normal in uncomplicated meningitis but often abnormal in herpes simplex encephalitis. It is often helpful in demonstrating complications of meningitis, such as subdural collections, hydrocephalus, or cerebral infarction.

7. In patients with suspected viral CNS infections, draw a

serum specimen acutely and save to compare with convalescent sera for rise in antibody titers.

8. In suspected enterovirus CNS infection (Coxsackie, Echo), stool specimen may be source of viral isolate. Mumps virus may be isolated from saliva, throat washing, or CSF.

9. Bacteremia is present in most patients with bacterial meningitis and should be detected by appropriate blood cultures.

10. Beware of coagulopathy in patients with fulminant meningitis (especially meningococcus).

11. PCR to identify herpes and tuberculosis is becoming available.

TREATMENT

Bacterial Meningitis

The mainstay of treatment of bacterial meningitis is intravenous antibiotics (see Table 22.1).
Other measures:

1. Patients with meningitis may develop cerebral swelling (edema). If this occurs, treatment with mannitol (0.25–0.50 gm/kg) and/or dexamethasone (10 mg IV then 4 mg every 6 hours.) may be given. Intubation and hyperventilation may be used to lower $PaCO_2$.

2. Seizures are common in meningitis and are usually treated with phenytoin.

3. Fluid restriction to 1200–1500 ml/day may be needed to reduce brain swelling or to control SIADH.

Viral Meningitis/Encephalitis

Treatment of viral CNS infection is primarily supportive and directed at possible complications. Apart from acyclovir, there is currently no specific antiviral therapy. Note:

1. Antiviral therapy for herpes simplex encephalitis with acyclovir has greatly improved morbidity and mortality. Usual dosage is 10 mg/kg every 8 hour IV.

2. Precautions in handling stool specimens are advised in

Table 22.1.
Antibiotics Used for Meningitis

Organism	Drug Used
Streptococcus pneumoniae	Penicillin G
Neisseria pneumoniae	Penicillin G
Haemophilus influenzae	Ampicillin and chloramphenicol until sensitivities return
Staphylococcus aureus	Naficillin ± rifampin or vancomycin for methicillin-resistant strains
Listeria monocytogenes	Ampicillin
Escherichia coli, Klebsiella	Cefotaxim
Proteus (unknown etiology above 8 years)	Penicillin or ampicillin

Dosages (per day in divided doses)	
Penicillin	24 million units
Ampicillin	12 gm
Chloramphenicol	4 gm
Naficillin	10–12 gm
Cefotaxin	12 gm
Vancomycin	2 gm

those with enteroviral infection.
3. Isolate patients suspected of having measles, chickenpox, or rubella.
4. Treat hyperthermia with acetaminophen or aspirin or cooling blanket.
5. Treat seizures that accompany encephalitis (phenytoin).

Fungal Meningitis

Cryptococcal meningitis is treated with amphotericin, with or without flucytosine. Follow renal functions carefully with these nephrotoxic drugs.

BRAIN ABSCESS

For a full discussion of brain abscess, please see Chapter 19 in (*Pediatric Neurology for the House Officer.*) If brain abscess is a serious consideration, avoid LP until mass lesion due to abscess has been excluded by CT or MRI.

Suggested Readings

Halperin JJ. Nervous system manifestations of Lyme disease. Rheumatic Dis Clin North Am 1989;15:635–647.

Jones R, Siekert RG. Neurological manifestations of infective endocarditis. Brain 1989;112:1295–1315.

Price RW. Viral infections of the nervous system. In: Cecil's textbook of medicine. Philadelphia: WB Saunders, 1988:sec.9.

Roos KL, Scheld WM. The management of fulminant meningitis in the intensive care unit. Infect Dis Clin North Am 1989;3:137–154.

Scheld WM, Wispelney B, eds. Meningitis. Infect Dis Clin North Am 1990;4(4).

Swartz MN. Bacterial meningitis. In: Cecil's textbook of medicine. Philadelphia, WB Saunders, 1988:ch.272–274.

Tunkel AR, Wispelney B, Scheld WM. Bacterial meningitis: recent advances in pathophysiology and treatment. Ann Intern Med 1990;112:610–623.

Weiner HL, Urion DK, Levitt LP. Pediatric neurology for the house officer. 3rd ed. Baltimore: Williams & Wilkins, 1988.

Whitley RJ. Herpes simplex virus infections of the control nervous system. Am J Med 1988;85(2A):61–67.

Chapter 23

AIDS and the Nervous System

The acquired immune deficiency syndrome (AIDS) is commonly associated with neurologic dysfunction. This is due to (*a*)
direct infection of the nervous system, (*b*) secondary opportunistic infections of the nervous system, *(c)* tumors associated
with AIDS, and (*d*) triggering of other processes such as inflammatory demyelinating peripheral neuropathies. No part of the
nervous system is spared in patients with human immunodeficiency virus (HIV) infection. The goal of the physician is to suspect and identify HIV infection in patients with a variety of nervous system conditions and to treat secondary infections accordingly.

BRAIN

1. *AIDS dementia complex.* Although many CNS manifestations
   of AIDS relate to secondary infections or tumors, the AIDS
   dementia complex represents a specific clinical entity most
   likely caused by direct brain infection by HIV virus. Note
   the following:
   a. Most AIDS patients are eventually afflicted with the
      AIDS dementia complex. Most commonly, the AIDS
      dementia complex develops after overt AIDS, although
      in many patients the dementia can present at the same
      time or before other manifestations of AIDS. In a small
      number of patients, dementia may be the only clinical
      sign of HIV infection prior to death.
   b. The onset of dementia is usually insidious, although

Table 23.1.
Neurologic Complications in HIV-1-Infected Patients[a]

BRAIN
  Predominantly nonfocal
    Aids dementia complex
    Cytomegalovirus (CMV) encephalitis
    Metabolic encephalopathies
    Herpes simplex virus (HSV) encephalitis
    Acute HIV-1 related encephalitis
  Predominantly focal
    Cerebral toxoplasmosis
    Primary CNS lymphoma
    Progressive multifocal leukoencepalopathy (PML)
    Cryptococcoma
    Varicella zoster virus (VZV) encephalitis
    Tuberculous brain abscess/tuberculoma
    Neurosyphilis (meningovascular)
    Vascular disorders

SPINAL CORD
  Vacuolar myelopathy
  Herpes zoster myelitis
  HSV myelitis

MENINGES
  Aseptic meningitis (HIV-1)
  Cryptococcal meningitis
  Metastatic lymphomatous meningitis
  Tuberculous meningitis
  Syphilitic meningitis

PERIPHERAL NERVE AND ROOT
  Infectious
    Herpes zoster
    CMV polyradiculopathy
  Virus or immune related
    Acute and chronic inflammatory demyelinating neuropathy
    Mononeuropathy
    Mononeuritis multiplex
    Autonomic neuropathy
    Sensorimotor polyneuropathy
    Distal painful sensory neuropathy
  Muscle
    Polymyositis and other myopathies

[a]   Adapted from Brew BJ, Sidtis JJ, Petito CK, Price RW. TThe neurologic complications of AIDS and human immunodeficiency virus infection. In: Plum F, ed. Advances in contemporary neurology. Philadelphia: FA Davis, 1988.

Table 23.2.
Timing of the Nervous System Complications of HIV-1 Infection in Relation to Stage of Systematic Disease[a]

	Systematic Disease Stage			
	Early	Latent	Early-Late	Late
CENTRAL NERVOUS SYSTEM				
Acute encephalitis	+			
Aseptic meningitis	+	+	+	+
AIDS dementia complex			+	+
Asymptomatic infection	+	+	+	+
Opportunistic CNS infections				+
Primary CNS lymphoma				+
Metastatic systemic lymphoma			+	+
PERIPHERAL NERVOUS SYSTEM				
Acute demyelinating polyneuropathy	+	+	+	
Chronic demyelinating polyneuropathy		+	+	
Mononeuropathies[b]	+			+
Mononeuropathy multiplex				+
Autonomic neuropathy				+
Sensorimotor polyneuropathy		+	+	+
Distal painful sensory neuropathy				+
MUSCLE				
Noninflammatory myopathy		+	+	+
Polymyostis		+	+	+

[a] Adapted from Brew BJ, Sidtis JJ, Petito CK, Price RW. TThe neurologic complications of AIDS and human immunodeficiency virus infection. In: Plum F, ed. Advances in contemporary neurology. Philadelphia: FA Davis, 1988.
[b] Excludes those with aseptic meningitis, lymphoma, herpes zoster, etc.

some patients may experience an abrupt, rapid worsening of their condition when the dementia appears suddenly over several days. In some patients, a rapidly accelerating dementia may occur in association with systemic illness.

c. Early symptoms and signs include cognitive changes (including forgetfulness and loss of concentration), motor difficulties (ataxia, leg weakness, deteriorating handwriting), behavioral abnormalities (apathy, psychosis), and other findings such as headache and seizures.

d. The late manifestations include severe dementia, ataxia, motor weakness, incontinence, tremor, and frontal release signs (suck, forced grasp).

e. Some patients may have an associated retinopathy, myelopathy, or peripheral neuropathy.

f. *Laboratory studies.* Patients have positive HIV serology and may have decreased CD4:CD8 T cell ratios in peripheral blood. Cerebrospinal fluid is abnormal in approximately half of patients and includes elevated protein levels, pleocytosis, and oligoclonal bands. CT and MRI scans are essential to rule out other focal conditions associated with AIDS (described below). Other findings include atrophy, enlargement of cortical sulci, enlarged ventricles, and white matter abnormalities. The EEG is usually normal in early stages of AIDS dementia complex.

g. Pathologically the AIDS dementia complex appears to involve subcortical white matter, thalamus and basal ganglia with relative sparing of the cerebral cortex.

h. Exclude metabolic drug encephalopathy, cryptococcal meningitis, tuberculosis, intracranial mass lesion, and neurosyphilis.

2. *Cerebral toxoplasmosis.* Cerebral toxoplasmosis is the commonest cause of focal brain pathology (intracranial mass lesion) in AIDS patients. It is particularly important to recognize early as prompt initiation of therapy can ameliorate the neurologic deficit. Note the following:

a. Approximately 15 to 30% of autopsied AIDS patients are positive for cerebral toxoplasmosis.

b. *Presenting clinical symptoms* and signs include focal manifestations, most commonly hemiparesis. In addition, patients may have seizures, aphasia, cranial nerve palsies, and ataxia. The most common nonfocal manifestations are confusion, lethargy, and headache.

c. *Laboratory studies.* The most sensitive studies include MRI or CT scan and blood serology. Contrast-enhancing ring lesions are seen on CT scan, and the MRI is quite sensitive in detecting *Toxoplasma* abscesses.

d. *Treatment.* Most patients respond to treatment with pyrimethamine (25 mg daily) and sulfadiazine (1 gm every 6 hours) if treated early. *NOTE:* Many patients with CNS toxoplasmosis may have underlying AIDS dementia. Thus, after resolution of the parasitic lesions, neurologic status may not return to normal.

e. Because cerebral toxoplasmosis is one of the more treatable neurologic complications of AIDS, a therapeutic trial for toxoplasmosis rather than a brain biopsy is indicated first.

f. The other major cause of intracranial mass lesion in AIDS is lymphoma. In many instances it may not be possible to distinguish toxoplasmosis from lymphoma without a biopsy.

3. *Other CNS infections.* A variety of other infections can affect the brain in AIDS patients. These include both viral and nonviral infections.

a. *Viral infections* include herpes simplex encephalitis, progressive multifocal leukoencephalopathy (caused by a papovavirus), cytomegalic virus encephalitis, and either HIV or CMV retinitis. CMV retinitis can rapidly cause blindness and can be treated with gancyclovir.

b. *Nonviral infections* include tuberculosis and fungal infections such as *Candida* and *Cryptococcus*.

4. *Neoplasms* also affect the brain in patients with AIDS: primary CNS lymphoma, systemic lymphoma with CNS involvement, and rarely, Kaposi's sarcoma. Lymphoma is treated with radiation therapy and corticosteroids.

5. *Stroke.* In some patients cerebrovascular accidents occur. Infarction and/or hemorrhage may occur. Hemorrhage may be associated with CNS lymphoma, infarction may be associated with arteritis, endocarditis, or tuberculous vasculopathy.

LEPTOMENINGES

1. The leptomeninges are frequently involved in AIDS. Examples include cryptococcal meningitis, aseptic meningitis, and lymphomatous meningitis. Diagnosis is carried out via spinal tap and appropriate culture of fluids, including checking for cryptococcal antigen.
2. Acute "aseptic" meningitis with headache, meningismus, cranial nerve palsies, and fever occurs at the time of seroconversion and probably represents primary infection with HIV. This process is generally self-limited. In some instances, a more indolent form of HIV-related meningitis occurs, presenting only as headache and low-grade pleocytosis.

SPINAL CORD

1. Spinal cord involvement in AIDS includes vacuolar myelopathy and viral myelitis that can be associated with a number of viruses, including herpes simplex virus, herpes zoster, and cytomegalic virus. These viral syndromes present as spinal cord dysfunction (e.g., leg weakness and incontinence) with cells in the spinal fluid.
2. *Myelopathy associated with HTLV-I virus.* A separate syndrome associated with HTLV-I virus affects the spinal cord. It is not related to HIV infection, but is associated with another retrovirus, HTLV-I. This entity is termed tropical spastic paraparesis (TSP) or the HAM syndrome (HTLV-I-associated myelopathy). The HAM syndrome is endemic in southern Japan. Clinically these patients have upper motor neuron spinal cord dysfunction with mild sensory and bladder disturbances. Diagnosis is based on high antibody titers to HTLV-I virus in serum and spinal fluid. The cause of nervous system dysfunction is not clear. Treatment with steroids may be of temporary benefit.

PERIPHERAL NERVES

1. Peripheral nerve involvement may take the form of inflammatory demyelinating polyneuropathy, sensorimotor peripheral neuropathy, mononeuropathy multiplex, and autonomic neuropathy.

2. Sensory neuropathy is seen in about 30% of patients. Symptoms include painful paresthesias affecting distal extremities. Symptoms occur late in the course of HIV infection. Treatment is symptomatic with drugs such as amitriptyline and carbamazepine. Etiology is unclear and may relate to HIV infection of dorsal root ganglia plus nutritional and toxic factors.

3. The inflammatory neuropathy may be either chronic or acute (Guillain-Barré syndrome). In addition to raised CSF protein, these patients have significant CSF pleocytosis generally not seen in Guillain-Barré. Patients respond to treatment with steroids or plasma exchange. Since plasma exchange is an accepted form of therapy for acute inflammatory polyneuropathy, all patients with this condition should be tested for AIDS.

4. Mononeuropathies may be seen in HIV infection in association with the AIDS-related complex.

5. Five to 10% of patients with HIV infection will develop herpes zoster nerve root infection (radiculitis). A characteristic dermatomal rash is often diagnostic. Treatment with acyclovir is recommended.

6. Newer drugs used to treat AIDS such as DDI, a purine analog, DDC, a pyrimidine analog, may cause a dose-related peripheral neuropathy.

MUSCLE

Myositis has been described as a rare complication of HIV infection. Muscle biopsies have shown inflammatory changes including multinucleated giant cells plus HIV antigens in the muscle. Treatment with steroids may be helpful.

Suggested Readings

Brew BJ, Sidtis JJ, Petito CK, Price RW. The neurologic complications of AIDS and human immunodeficiency virus infection. In Advances in Contemporary Neurology. Plum F. ed. Philadelphia: FA Davis, 1988.

Bridge TP, Ingraham LJ. Central nervous system effects of human immunodeficiency virus type I. Annu Rev Med 1990;41:159–168.

Cornblath DR, McArthur JC, Kennedy PGE, Witte AS, Griffin JW. Inflammatory demyelinating peripheral neuropathies associated with human T-cell lymphotropic virus type III infection. Ann Neurol 1987;21:32.

de Gans J, Portegies P. Neurological complications of infection with human immunodeficiency virus type I. Clin Neurol Neurosurg 1989;91(3):199–219.

Kieburtz K, Schiffer RB. Neurologic manifestations of human immunodeficiency virus infections. Neurol Clin 1989;7:447–468.

Lange DJ, Britton CB, Younger DS, Hays AP. The neuromuscular manifestations of human immunodeficiency virus infections. Arch Neurol 1988;45:1084.

Levy RM, Bredesen DE, Rosenblum ML. Neurologic manifestations of the acquired immunodeficiency syndrome (AIDS): experience at UCSF and review of the literature. J Neurosurg 1985;62:475.

McArthur JC. Neurologic manifestation of AIDS. Medicine 1987;66:407.

Navia BA, Jordan BD, Price RW. The AIDS dementia complex I. Clinical features. Ann Neurol 1986;19:517.

Chapter 24

Neurology of Uremia

MENTAL STATUS CHANGES

One of the most common features of renal failure is an altered mental status. It may range from irritability and difficulty in concentration (e.g., performing "serial 7s") to actual psychotic reactions. Mental status changes in uremia fluctuate; periods of confusion are interspersed with periods of lucidity.

Acute changes in mental status are generally encountered postdiuresis or postdialysis when there have been rapid electrolyte shifts, even though actual electrolyte values are improved ("dysequilibrium syndrome"). Metabolically, brain shifts of urea and/or pH lag or often do not parallel systemic changes. Slowly developing renal failure causes fewer status changes than does rapidly developing failure.

EEG changes are usual with an altered mental status and usually parallel the degree of metabolic encephalopathy. Most patients with a blood urea nitrogen level above 60 mg/100 ml have EEG abnormalities (generalized slowing).

Although most mental status changes (increased irritability and lack of ability to concentrate in the "stable uremic" or periods of marked disorientation secondary to rapid metabolic shifts) are not secondary to treatable nervous system disease, keep other possibilities in mind:

1. *Infection.* Fungal or other uncommon CNS pathogens are not uncommon in uremics. Perform a lumbar puncture when there is unexplained confusion or fever in the uremic patient after performing a CT scan or MRI to rule out sub-

dural hematoma. Remember to do an India ink preparation for *Cryptococcus* or test for cryptococcal antigen if there are cells in the CSF (see Chapter 29).

2. *Subdural hematoma.* Uremics have an increased bleeding tendency, and subdural collections may develop with mild head trauma or during dialysis. If a subdural hematoma is suspected because of lateralizing signs or persistent lethargy with headache, obtain a CT scan or MRI.

CONVULSIONS

Convulsions are a common feature of renal disease; they signify different processes, depending on the type (generalized or focal) and the clinical setting (e.g., postdialysis). Patients with *acute anuria* may develop convulsions on the 8th to 11th day of renal failure or with the onset of diuresis and subsequent rapid electrolyte shifts. These convulsions tend to be generalized.

Convulsions also appear late in the course of *chronic renal disease* and frequently are associated with abnormal blood chemistries: acidosis, hypokalemia, and hyponatremia. No one abnormal electrolyte is consistently associated with seizures, but the greater the potassium/calcium ratio, the greater is the risk of convulsion.

Seizures are common *postdialysis.*

In patients with either acute or chronic renal failure, the first convulsion may be a *preterminal* event.

Treatment of Convulsions

1. The drug of choice is *phenytoin,* which is metabolized by the liver, not kidney, and is not removed during dialysis. Administer 1000 mg (15 mg/kg) IV over 30–45 minutes if immediate therapeutic levels are needed, then 300 to 400 mg daily. Follow the phenytoin levels, including the free (unbound) phenytoin level, which is increased in renal failure (see Chapter 11).

2. *Generalized or multifocal* seizures (one side then the other) occurring during metabolic flux (dialysis, diuresis) are generally self-limited. Treat with phenytoin. When the patient's condition has stabilized, anticonvulsants may be withdrawn.

3. Patients with persistent *focal* seizures should be worked up

in search of subdural hematoma, tumor, infection, or infarct with CT scan or MRI, LP, and EEG. Patients may have tiny areas of cortical hemorrhage that account for focal seizures.

4. Check for predisposing electrolyte disturbances and correct where appropriate.
5. Some physicians give phenytoin prophylactically to patients who are about to experience rapid electrolyte shifts (e.g., during dialysis).

PERIPHERAL NEUROPATHY

Early. Patients often begin with a "restless leg syndrome." The leg feels uncomfortable when the patient is still and relief occurs after ambulation. Another early neuropathic syndrome consists of painful, burning paresthesias of the feet similar to those seen in alcoholics and associated with dietary insufficiency. Resolution may follow proper diet and vitamin supplements.

Late. A more severe peripheral neuropathy develops over weeks to months and is not diet-dependent. Check for distal loss of all sensory modalities (pinprick, position, vibration). The legs are affected significantly more than the arms. The neuropathy is both motor and sensory and may lead to actual paraplegia (at this stage the arms may also become involved). Treatment is extremely difficult. Although dialysis helps somewhat, it is generally ineffective; renal transplantation reverses the neuropathy. Nerve conduction velocities are slow in most uremics, regardless of whether they have symptomatic neuropathy.

OTHER NEUROLOGIC FEATURES OF UREMIA

Dialysis may precipitate convulsions or a toxic encephalopathy. In this "reverse urea syndrome," urea leaves the brain more slowly than it leaves the blood; fluid is thus drawn into the brain, resulting in acute swelling. There may also be a lag in pH equilibrium. The encephalopathy usually clears in 24–48 hours. Remember, subdural hematoma sometimes follows dialysis.

Asterixis frequently accompanies uremic encephalopathy, as do muscle fasciculations and myoclonus.

Muscle cramps may occur and generally are not related to a specific electrolyte abnormality, although they are more frequent when water intoxication is present. Chvostek's sign may be positive in uremia; it is correlated with the acidosis and elevated potassium/calcium ratio rather than with decreased calcium alone. There may be mild proximal muscle weakness.

"Uremic amaurosis" has been reported with the acute development of blindness; this may be related to focal cerebral edema. Complete recovery usually occurs.

Cerebral emboli may occur during the declotting of shunts used for hemodialysis.

Dialysis dementia has been reported in patients with uremia; it represents a progressive neurologic deterioration in patients on hemodialysis. It consists of dementia, myoclonus, speech disorders, neuropsychiatric abnormalities, gait abnormalities, and EEG changes. Etiology is unknown; some cases may be due to metal (aluminum) intoxication, but in most cases the etiology is obscure. Clinical and EEG improvement may follow treatment with diazepam or other anticonvulsants.

Cranial nerve abnormalities in uremia may cause nystagmus, facial weakness, dizziness, and hearing loss. Symptoms due to the uremia must be differentiated from those due to ototoxic/nephrotoxic drugs.

Carpal tunnel syndrome is more common in patients on hemodialysis.

TABLE 24.1.
Signs and Symptoms of Uremic Encephalopathy[a]

Early	Moderate	Severe
Anorexia	Vomiting	Itching
Nausea	Sluggishness	Disorientation
Insomnia	Easy fatigue	Confusion
Restlessness	Drowsiness	Bizarre behavior
Decreased attention span	Sleep inversion	Slurring of speech
Inability to manage ideas	Volatile emotions	Hypothermia
Decreased sexual interest	Paranoia	Myoclonus
	Decreased cognitive function	Asterixis
	Inability to decipher abstractions	Convulsions
	Decreased sexual performance	Stupor
		Coma

[a] From: Fraser CL, Arieff AI. Nervous system complications of uremia. Ann Intern Med 1988; 109:143–153. With permission.

Transplant patients being treated with *cyclosporine* may experience tremors and paresthesias early after transplantation, related to high-dose cyclosporine: this usually resolves when the cyclosporine dose is decreased.

Some patients treated for *transplant rejection* with *OKT3* monoclonal antibody may experience an aseptic meningitis syndrome (headaches, stiff neck) with pleocytosis in the CSF, related to the monoclonal antibody. If CSF culture is negative, no treatment is needed.

Suggested Readings

Bruno A, Adams HP. Neurologic problems in renal transplant recipients. Neurol Clin 1989;7:617–627.

Fraser CL, Arieff AI. Nervous system complications in uremia. Ann Intern Med 1988;109:143.

Lazaro RP, Kirshner HS. Proximal muscle weakness in uremia. Case reports and review of the literature. Arch Neurol 1980;37:555.

Lockwood AH. Neurologic complications of renal disease. Neurol Clin 1988;6:305.

Raskin NH, Fishman RA. Neurologic disorders in renal failure. N Engl J Med 1976;294:143.

Chapter 25

Neurology of Alcoholism

SEIZURES

Seizures are common in the alcoholic and represent at least two different phenomena. It is important to distinguish the two types of "alcoholic seizures" because treatment and workup are different.

[handwritten annotations: Inter-ictal → normal EEG; "Rum Fits" → Generalized 2° to w/D]

"Rum fits" are brief, self-limited, generalized seizures secondary to abstinence from alcohol or a reduction in the usual intake. They do not represent a true convulsive disorder, and most occur 12–48 hours earlier or later (rarely after 96 hours). A night's sleep without alcohol may be enough to precipitate a seizure. Remember, rum fits can occur in the "businessman-drinker" who comes to the hospital for another reason. Alcohol withdrawal seizures tend to appear in groups of two or three and then stop. The patient is usually tremulous and jittery. The interictal EEG in these patients is normal, and if the history is characteristic, the patient requires no further neurologic workup or anticonvulsant medication. Often a patient is placed on anticonvulsants in the hospital after the first seizure, but when it becomes apparent that it was a "withdrawal seizure," anticonvulsants are tapered and discontinued. Patients with rum fits are markedly sensitive to photic stimulation during EEG. They are also at a higher risk for developing delirium tremens.

Seizures Precipitated by Alcohol — Focal (intrinsic lesion)

Abnormal EEG

These alcohol-induced seizures are usually focal and reflect an intrinsic CNS lesion. Seizures of this type may occur during the period of intoxication. Such patients generally have an abnormal EEG; they require a basic neurologic workup for seizure and treatment with anticonvulsants. Focal seizures in the alcoholic often represent posttraumatic epilepsy due to multiple falls. It is important to remember that focal seizures represent CNS pathology, and alcoholics are especially prone to subdural hematoma and meningitis. Persistently focal seizures in an alcoholic should be considered to be caused by a subdural hematoma until proven otherwise. Of course, alcoholics have the same risk for brain tumor as does the general population.

Was the seizure focal or generalized? When did it occur?

Remember the questions to answer when treating the seizure of an alcoholic: Was the seizure focal or generalized? When did it occur in relation to drinking?

ALCOHOLIC TREMULOUSNESS—DELIRIUM TREMENS

The spectrum of alcohol withdrawal symptoms ranges from mild tremulousness to fatal delirium tremens (DTs). The underlying physiology in these states is related to abstinence from alcohol, not to specific dietary or vitamin insufficiency. Similar withdrawal states can occur after stopping other CNS depressants (e.g., barbiturates, diazepam). DTs and withdrawal seizures can be produced in normal individuals on good diets who are placed on large amounts of alcohol and then withdrawn. Seizures are a point on the spectrum of withdrawal symptomatology. An alcoholic who stops drinking is subject to the following:

1. *Tremulousness* is one of the first signs of alcohol withdrawal, beginning approximately 8 hours after cessation of drinking (often after a night's sleep) and reaching its peak at 24 hours. The patient is jittery, startles easily, and often shows a gross irregular tremor of the hands. Although these symptoms are most severe at 24 hours, it may take 7–10 days before the patient is back to normal. Drinkers who suffer

from tremulousness upon arising in the morning may take a drink to "calm their nerves."

2. *Seizures* (discussed above).

3. *Hallucinations* appear during the withdrawal period and are commonly visual, although they may be auditory. Sometimes the patient hallucinates in the presence of an otherwise clear sensorium.

4. *Delirium tremens* completes the spectrum. This reaction occurs about 72–96 hours after cessation of drinking. Those who have had a chronic period of drinking before cessation experience the most severe form of DTs. They suffer from tremulousness, hallucinations, and marked autonomic hyperactivity (tachycardia, hyperhidrosis, fever, dilated pupils). DTs are relatively uncommon sequelae of alcoholic withdrawal, but can be fatal; they are often preceded by an alcoholic withdrawal seizure.

Treatment of DTs

Treatment consists of supportive care. Adequate diet and vitamins have no effect on the course of alcohol withdrawal, but must be given to prevent other complications. Pay careful attention to fluid and electrolyte balance, and search thoroughly for underlying disease (e.g., subdural hematoma, pneumonia, or meningitis). These diseases are not uncommon and often are the factors that make DTs fatal. We use chlordiazepoxide (Librium), 50 mg orally every 4–6 hours (the initial dose may be given IV), or paraldehyde, 10 ml orally or rectally every 4–6 hours, to lessen the agitation (watch for oversedation). Some use diazepam 25–50 mg orally four times a day. Diazepam may be given in small intravenous doses (2.5 mg or 5 mg). Serax, 10–15 mg, 3–4/day may be better metabolized by patients with liver problems. There is no evidence that steroids are of benefit. Atenolol, a β-adrenergic blocker, is sometimes helpful in selected patients with the alcohol withdrawal syndrome. It may not be possible to prevent DTs, but one can lessen the severity of agitation with medication; by controlling fluid and electrolyte balance, the chances for recovery are good.

VITAMIN DEFICIENCY SYNDROMES AND ALCOHOLISM

In addition to the alcohol withdrawal syndrome, there is a group of vitamin deficiency syndromes seen almost exclusively in alcoholics. (They also appear in nonalcoholics with poor diets.)

Wernicke's Encephalopathy

Wernickes
Confusion
ophthalmoplegia
Ataxia
Thiamine

This thiamine deficiency syndrome consists of a characteristic clinical triad:

1. *Ocular changes.* Look for nystagmus on horizontal and/or vertical gaze, sixth nerve palsies that are generally bilateral, and paralysis of conjugate gaze. In severe forms there may be total ophthalmoplegia.
2. *Gait difficulties.* Check for ataxia: a wide-based gait, falling, or inability to walk or stand.
3. *Mental symptoms.* Patients usually manifest a quiet confusional state. *Korsakoff's psychosis* is an extension of the mental symptoms of Wernicke's disease and becomes apparent later if the Wernicke's syndrome is untreated. The main feature is a marked disorder of memory and confabulation. The patient is unable to learn new material such as the doctor's name or who visited 10 minutes earlier. CT scans in chronic alcoholics often show evidence of cerebral and cerebellar atrophy.

Korsakoffs
Retrograde amnesia
anterograde
Confabulation
Korsakoff

In addition to the above triad, thiamine deficiency can produce dysautonomia, including cardiac failure and ECG changes.

Treatment consists of thiamine (50 mg IV and 50 mg IM) to improve the oculomotor dysfunction and to prevent the development of Korsakoff's psychosis. GI malabsorption in alcoholics makes oral treatment unreliable. The 50 mg IM dose should be repeated daily until the patient resumes a normal diet. Occasionally, larger doses may be needed initially to improve oculomotor dysfunction. Be careful when giving intravenous fluids to alcoholics; glucose may cause depletion of thiamine stores and precipitate Wernicke's syndrome (add thiamine to the intravenous solution).

In alcoholics: add thiamine to intravenous solutions.

Wernicke's syndrome can also occur in nonalcoholics who depend on parenteral alimentation for several days (e.g., surgical or burn unit patients) or in patients with malnutrition due to starvation, renal failure, cancer, or AIDS.

Polyneuropathy

Polyneuropathy occurs in alcoholics secondary to nutritional factors and may also be related in part to the toxic effects of alcohol. Most patients are asymptomatic but lose ankle and sometimes knee jerks. When symptoms occur, they consist of burning feet, pain, paresthesia, and mild distal weakness. The feet may be so sensitive that bed covers touching the feet are painful. In severe cases the weakness may progress to wrist-drop and foot-drop. Polyneuropathy and Wernicke's syndrome often occur in the same patient.

Treatment consists of improving the diet, complete abstinence from alcohol, and adding vitamin supplements. Some clinicians give phenytoin or carbamazepine during the acute stage; recovery is slow but usually occurs with abstinence and proper diet.

OTHER NEUROLOGIC COMPLICATIONS OF ALCOHOLISM

Cerebellar degeneration affects men more frequently than women, and midline structures more than cerebellar hemispheres. Thus, there is a wide-based gait with truncal instability and a less prominent limb ataxia. The symptoms appear over weeks to months, although they may come on acutely. The acutely occurring syndrome has a better prognosis and may not represent actual cerebellar structural damage, as does the chronic form. Treatment consists of dietary and vitamin support. Further abstinence from alcohol is crucial.

Some patients may have slowly developing myopathy with *proximal muscle weakness,* often in conjunction with alcoholic cardiac myopathy. There is an acute form with muscle pain, weakness, and elevated creatinine phosphokinase and myoglobinuria. Treatment is symptomatic.

Rare complications of alcoholism or malnutrition include

central pontine myelinolysis and the Marchiafava-Bignami corpus callosum syndrome.

Suggested Readings

Charness ME, Simon RP, Greenberg DA. Ethanol and the nervous system. N Engl J Med 1989;321:442–454.

Kraus ML. Randomized clinical trial of atenolol in patients with alcohol withdrawal. N Engl J Med 1985;313:905.

Reuter JB. Wernicke's encephalopathy. N Engl J Med 1985;312:1035.

Simon PP. Alcohol and seizures. N Engl J Med 1988;319:715.

Victor M, Adams R, Collins G. The Wernicke-Korsakoff syndrome Philadelphia: FA Davis, 1971.

Chapter 26

Neurology of Other Systemic Diseases

Most systemic diseases exhibit neurologic manifestations, as described in preceding chapters on the neurology of diabetes, malignancy, uremia, and alcohol. The physician must recognize the large variety of neurologic complications that accompany systemic disorders and treat them accordingly.

CARDIAC DISEASE

Cardiac abnormalities can cause either reduced cerebral perfusion or emboli that lead to neurologic sequelae. The severity of neurologic manifestations of reduced cardiac output varies with the rate and extent of decreased cerebral perfusion. Ischemic brain injury can lead to seizures, cerebral edema, loss of consciousness, amnesia, and dementia.

Emboli from the heart are the cause of 15% of ischemic strokes. Thrombi, from which emboli emerge, may develop from a left atrial or ventricular mural thrombus, an intracardiac tumor, bacterial and nonbacterial endocarditis, or from the systemic and right heart circulation via intracardiac shunts (paradoxical emboli). Conditions that predispose the patient to develop such emboli include atrial fibrillation, acute and chronic ischemic heart disease, and valvular heart disease (rheumatic and prosthetic). Mitral annulus calcification, calcific aortic stenosis, and atrial septal aneurysm can also cause cerebral emboli.

Hemorrhagic strokes may occur following an occluding embolus and result from reperfusion of tissue infarcted by the embolus. Young patients without evidence of cerebrovascular disease should be suspected of having a cardiac cause of stroke. Electrocardiogram, echocardiography, prolonged ECG monitoring to identify arrhythmias, transesophageal echocardiography, and isotope-labeled platelet scintigraphy are helpful tests for detecting the cause of cardiogenic stroke.

Anticoagulation therapy reduces the risk of embolism in atrial fibrillation, rheumatic mitral stenosis, and cardiomyopathy with ventricular thrombi. Following an MI, patients are at risk for stroke, especially with anterior wall infarction. If echocardiography detects a developing thrombus, anticoagulation reduces the risk of post-MI stroke by at least 60%.

ENDOCRINE DISEASE

1. <u>Thyroid.</u> *Hyperthyroid* patients often complain of nervousness, fatigue, and irritability. They may have seizures, tremor, and chorea, and usually have brisk tendon reflexes. They may also develop ophthalmopathy including proptosis and ophthalmoplegia; myopathy with proximal muscle weakness and wasting is common. *Hypothyroid* patients complain of fatigue and exhibit apathy, decreased attention, and slowness in answering questions. Myxedema coma is rare and carries a high mortality rate. Some patients may develop seizures, obstructive sleep apnea, ataxia, or sensorineural hearing loss. Myopathy is common, including exertional pain, stiffness, and cramps. CPK is usually elevated. On physical examination, increased reflex relaxation time can usually be demonstrated.

2. <u>Parathyroid.</u> Patients with *hyperparathyroidism* often display psychiatric symptoms such as those associated with mania, schizophrenia, or depression. Myopathy is common. Patients with *hypoparathyroidism* may have psychiatric symptoms similar to those seen in hyperparathyroidism, and seizures can occur from hypocalcemia, particularly in hyperparathyroid patients after adenoma removal. Hypocalcemia and hypomagnesemia can cause tetany. To elicit latent tetany, have the patient hyperventilate and tap the facial nerve, causing facial muscle contraction (Chvostek's sign), or occlude venous return from an arm, resulting in carpopedal spasm (Trousseau's sign).

3. <u>Glucocorticoid.</u> Myopathy is common with corticosteroid therapy, and myalgia may accompany the weakness. Treatment involves tapering or use of alternate-day steroids, alternate forms of immunosuppression, or nonfluorinated steroids. Patients with Cushing's syndrome may experience psychiatric symptoms. Patients with Addison's disease, following withdrawal from steroids, may experience acute confusional states or psychosis. Seizures can occur from hyponatremia.

FLUID AND ELECTROLYTE DISTURBANCES

1. <u>Sodium.</u> Manifestations of *hyponatremia* range from confusion to coma. Patients may also experience convulsions, hemiparesis, ataxia, tremor, aphasia, and corticospinal tract signs. Sodium must be corrected rapidly to 120–125 mEq/liter when convulsions are present, because such patients have a high mortality. However, too rapid correction of hyponatremia may result in central pontine myelinosis. Patients with subarachnoid hemorrhage and hyponatremia should not be fluid restricted, as their hyponatremia, previously attributed to SIADH, is usually associated with volume depletion. *Hypernatremia* causes symptoms from lethargy to coma, seizures, rigidity, tremor, myoclonus, asterixis, and chorea. It may be seen in association with fluid loss and in the elderly from dehydration. Hyperosmolar states may be associated with cerebral edema.

2. <u>Potassium.</u> *Hypokalemia* causes muscle weakness, myalgia, and fatigability. With very low potassium levels (less than 2.5 mEq/liter), rhabdomyolysis and myoglobinuria may occur. Rapid recovery occurs with potassium replacement. *Hyperkalemia* is cardiotoxic and is rarely associated with neurologic symptoms before the heart is affected.

3. <u>Calcium.</u> *Hypercalcemia* may occur in patients with malignant neoplasms (particularly breast and lung cancer and multiple myeloma) and in patients with hyperparathyroidism. Patients may experience lethargy, muscle weakness, fatigability, confusion, headache, convulsions, and even coma. *Hypocalcemia* is rare but can be seen in patients with renal failure. Acute hypocalcemia most often occurs following thyroid or parathyroid surgery and is a complication of

acute pancreatitis. Patients are agitated and may experience delirium, hallucinations, and psychosis. Seizures may occur.

4. <u>Magnesium.</u> With decreased calcium, patients are irritable and confused and may experience tetany, convulsions, tremor, and myoclonus. They are hyperreflexic and demonstrate a Chvostek sign. Treatment of convulsions is via parental magnesium. *Hypermagnesemia* is rare and occurs with increased intake in the setting of decreased renal function. It causes lethargy and confusion, and muscle paralysis may result.

GASTROINTESTINAL DISEASE

1. <u>Hepatic encephalopathy.</u> Mental changes range from delirium to coma. Tremor, paratonia, asterixis, and hyperactive reflexes are also seen. The EEG demonstrates slowing and triphasic waves and serum ammonia levels are increased. Causes of encephalopathy include toxins and metabolic derangements. If focal neurologic symptoms occur in the setting of hepatic encephalopathy, check for a structural lesion. Hepatic encephalopathy may unmask previously asymptomatic lesions such as a chronic subdural hematoma. Imaging may also demonstrate subarachnoid or intracerebral hemorrhage, related to coagulopathy associated with hepatic disease.

2. <u>Malabsorption.</u> A number of GI disorders are associated with malabsorption (e.g., inflammatory bowel disease, post–gastric resection). This may lead to thiamine deficiency and Wernicke's encephalopathy or Korsakoff's psychosis (Chapter 25). Cyanocobalamin (vitamin B_{12}) can be deficient in a vegetarian's diet, following gastric resection, with intrinsic factor deficiency (pernicious anemia), in a patient without a functional terminal ileum, and with pancreatic insufficiency. Patients experience paresthesias, sensory loss, ataxia, and dementia. Patients who lack vitamin B_6 can develop peripheral neuropathy. Those with vitamin A deficiency have an association with pseudotumor cerebri; inadequate amounts of vitamin E causes neuropathy and cerebellar disease.

3. <u>Other</u> <u>illnesses.</u> *Wilson's disease* is associated with cirrhosis and caudate-putamen degeneration. Patients may have

tremor, dysarthria, dementia, and psychiatric symptoms. Patients have a Kayser-Fleischer ring on ophthalmologic examination, decreased serum ceruloplasmin level, and increased copper concentration on liver biopsy.

Chronic hepatocerebral degeneration is a slowly progressive neurologic syndrome manifested by chronic intermittent episodes of hepatic encephalopathy seen in patients with hepatic disease. Permanent neurologic signs and symptoms may result, including tremor, ataxia, dysarthria, nystagmus, dementia, choreoathetosis, pyramidal tract signs, and grasp reflexes. Patients with portal-systemic shunts may experience a myelopathy associated with dysarthria. The etiology is unclear.

HEMATOLOGIC DISEASE

1. <u>Anemia.</u> Common symptoms include fatigue, headache, and lightheadedness. Individuals with sickle cell anemia may develop stroke, convulsions, or change in level of consciousness. Patients with chronic hematologic diseases characterized by bone marrow failure or hemolytic anemia have extramedullary hematopoiesis that may involve meninges surrounding the spinal cord and brain, leading to myelopathy or intracranial mass lesions.

2. <u>Hyperviscosity.</u> Patients may experience headache, lightheadedness, tinnitus, stupor, convulsions, or stroke. Causative diseases include polycythemia vera, leukocytosis, and paraproteinemias with Waldenstrom's macroglobulinemia and multiple myeloma. Leukemic patients have a high incidence of intracerebral hemorrhage, and paraproteinemic patients have reduced cerebral blood flow, peripheral neuropathies, mononeuritis multiplex, and cerebral infarction.

3. <u>Thrombocytopenia.</u> Immune thrombocytopenic purpura can follow viral infection, with an increased incidence of intracranial hemorrhage. Patients with thrombotic thrombocytopenic purpura (TTP) have prominent neurologic symptoms including headache, hemiparesis, aphasia, and seizures. Corticosteroids and plasma exchange may be of benefit.

4. <u>Hemophilia.</u> Patients are predisposed to develop intracranial hemorrhage, subdural hematoma, subarachnoid hemorrhage, and epidural hematoma of the spinal cord.

Peripheral neuropathies may develop secondary to compression by soft-tissue hemorrhage, particularly femoral neuropathy from retroperitoneal bleeding. These bleeding complications may also occur in patients on anticoagulation therapy.

NOTE: Antiphospholipid antibodies, including lupus anticoagulants and anticardiolipin antibodies, may be associated with focal cerebral ischemia and should be tested for in young patients with unexplained cerebral ischemic events.

PULMONARY DISEASE

1. <u>Respiratory insufficiency</u>. Hypoxia, hypercapnia, and respiratory acidosis may cause headache, mental status changes, motor disturbances, ocular abnormalities, and paresthesias. Twitching and tremor result from increased sympathetic nervous system activity. Asterixis, generalized seizures, and myoclonus may occur. Polycythemia from chronic respiratory insufficiency causes headache and dizziness.

2. <u>Hyperventilation</u>. Anxious individuals may have neurologic symptoms if they hyperventilate, including paresthesias, lightheadedness, altered consciousness, carpal spasm, muscle cramps, visual blurring, dyspnea, chest pain, and an elicitable Chvostek sign. Hyperventilation syndrome is usually psychogenic, but it may be associated with medication, alcohol withdrawal, or CNS lesions. Rebreathing into a paper bag at the first awareness of symptoms and β-blockers may be helpful.

RHEUMATOLOGIC DISEASES, SARCOIDOSIS, AND VASCULITIDES

1. <u>SLE.</u> One-half of lupus patients have neurologic manifestations, but most have an established diagnoses of SLE before neurologic manifestations develop. CNS lupus includes seizures, paresis, ataxia, chorea, scotomata, meningitis, cranial neuropathies, and optic neuritis. CNS lupus is usually treated with corticosteroids, cyclophosphamide, azathioprine, or plasmapheresis; CNS infections are more frequent

in lupus patients because of immunosuppressive therapy. Psychotropic medications may provide symptomatic relief of neuropsychiatric manifestations. The PNS is less frequently affected, but patients may have sensory and sensorimotor neuropathies, mononeuropathies, mononeuritis multiplex, and an acute ascending sensorimotor neuropathy similar to Guillain-Barré.

2. <u>Sjögren's disease.</u> Neurologic manifestations include seizures, movement disorders, psychiatric symptoms, aseptic meningitis, symptoms mimicking multiple sclerosis, and progressive dementia. PNS involvement (occurring in 25% of patients) includes polyneuropathy and neuropathies due to nerve entrapment. Spinal cord involvement includes progressive myelopathy, transverse myelopathy, Brown-Sequard syndrome, neurogenic bladder, and spinal subarachnoid hemorrhage. Sjögren's disease is also associated with neuromuscular disorders including myasthenia gravis, polymyositis, and inclusion body myositis. Treatment of CNS Sjögren's disease involves the use of steroids and/or cyclophosphamide.

3. <u>Rheumatoid arthritis (RA).</u> Neurologic manifestations most often occur in patients with long-standing disease and with positive rheumatoid factor. Neuropathy is common. Compression or entrapment neuropathy occurs when swollen tissues compress peripheral nerves. Most common is median nerve compression at the wrist (carpal tunnel syndrome). Distal sensory neuropathies with dysesthesia or burning in the hands or feet occur, but these symptoms are often difficult to distinguish from the accompanying arthritis. Sensorimotor neuropathy is less common, is progressive, and can be disabling. Myelopathy can also affect RA patients because the cervical spine is frequently involved and the cervical canal can become narrowed during neck flexion following atlantoaxial subluxation. Posterior circulation symptoms including vertigo and weakness can occur due to vertebral artery flow compromise by compression or thrombosis. Patients with advanced RA should wear cervical collars when driving or riding in a car and should have cervical spine films in flexion (provided there is no odontoid fracture) prior to undergoing general anesthesia. RA may also be associated with a myopathy.

4. <u>Osteoarthritis.</u> Spinal canal contents and spinal nerves may be compressed by osteoarthritis from intervertebral disc disease, spinal stenosis, and bony impingement, and peripheral nerves may become entrapped, all resulting in neurologic symptoms.

5. <u>Sarcoidosis.</u> Granulomas in the CNS can occur in extradural, subdural, leptomeningeal, and parenchymal locations, causing a wide spectrum of CNS symptoms that include (*a*) aseptic meningitis with headache, lethargy, vomiting, papilledema, and meningismus; (*b*) hydrocephalus secondary to granulomatous obstruction of CSF; (*c*) basilar meningitis affecting cranial nerves 7–12 and the optic nerve; (*d*) granulomas in the cerebral hemispheres, which can cause progressive dementia and epileptic foci. In sarcoidosis, hypercalcemia or opportunistic infections may also cause neurologic symptoms. CSF usually shows elevated protein, a mononuclear pleocytosis, and decreased glucose. Peripheral neuropathy with mononeuritis multiplex or slowly progressive symmetric sensorimotor neuropathy are also seen.

8. <u>Vasculitis.</u> CNS vasculitis may cause headache, behavioral changes, memory impairment, psychiatric symptoms, alteration in consciousness, and generalized seizures. Focal cerebral deficits with a stroke-like picture can be due to vasculitis and should be considered particularly in a young patient. Cranial nerve palsies may also occur. Neurologic symptoms may be the only manifestation of a systemic vasculitis.

In the PNS, mononeuritis multiplex and a distal symmetric "stocking glove" sensorimotor polyneuropathy may occur. Patients experience severe, burning dysesthetic pain in the distribution of the involved nerves. Painful focal neuropathies should suggest the possibility of vasculitis.

Patients may have an elevated ESR and CSF protein and lymphocytic pleocytosis in the CSF during active disease. MRI demonstrates small areas of cerebral infarction. However, a brain, meningeal, or peripheral nerve biopsy specimen is often necessary to make a definitive diagnosis of isolated CNS or PNS vasculitis. Treatment involves removing possible inciting antigens such as medications, infectious agents, or environmental toxins. Immunosuppressive therapy with corticosteroids and cytotoxic drugs (cyclophosphamide) is usually helpful.

Suggested Readings

Albers JW, Nostrant TT, Riggs JE. Neurologic manifestations of gastrointestinal disease. Neurol Clin 1989;7:525–548.

Brick JE, Brick JF. Neurologic manifestations of rheumatologic disease. Neurol Clin 1989;7:629–640.

Heck AW, Phillips LH. Sarcoidosis and the nervous system. Neurol Clin 1989;7:641–654.

Hietaharju A, Yli-Kerttula U, Hakkinen V, Frey H. Nervous system manifestations in Sjögren's syndrome. Acta Neurol Scand 1990;81:144–152.

Jozefowicz RF. Neurologic manifestations of pulmonary disease. Neurol Clin 1989;7:605–616.

Kaminski HJ, Ruff RL. Neurologic complications of endocrine diseases. Neurol Clin 1989;7:489–508.

Kissel JT. Neurologic manifestations of vasculitis. Neurol Clin 1989;7:655–674.

Levine SR, Deegan MJ, Futrell N, et al. Cerebrovascular and neurologic disease associated with antiphospholipid antibodies: 48 cases. Neurology 1990;40:1181–1189.

Massey EW, Riggs JE. Neurologic manifestations of hematologic disease. Neurol Clin 1989;7:549–562.

Moore PM. Diagnosis and management of isolated angiitis of the central nervous system. Neurology 1989;39:167–173.

Provost TT, Vasily D, Alexander E. Sjögren's syndrome; cutaneous, immunologic, and nervous system manifestations. Neurol Clin 1987;5:405–426.

Riggs JE. Neurologic manifestations of fluid and electrolyte disturbances. Neurol Clin 1989;7:509–524.

Riggs JE, ed. Neurologic manifestations of systemic disease. Vol. 7(3). Philadelphia: WB Saunders, 1989.

Rothstein JD, Herlong HF. Neurologic manifestations of hepatic disease. Neurol Clin 1989;7:563–578.

Sherman DG, Helgason CM. Neurologic manifestations of cardiac disease. Neurol Clin 1989;7:469–488.

Sigal LH. The neurologic presentations of vasculitis and rheumatologic syndromes. Medicine 1987;66:157.

Stremmel W, Meyerrose KW, Miederau C, et al. Wilson's disease: clinical presentation, treatment, and survival. Ann Intern Med 1991;115:720–726.

Wolf PA, Abbott RD, Kannel WB. Atrial fibrillation as an independent risk factor for stroke: the Framingham Study. Stroke 1991;22:983–988.

Chapter 27

Raised Intracranial Pressure

Raised intracranial pressure may be secondary to a focal mass lesion or more diffuse processes. *Signs* and *symptoms* include headache, nausea and vomiting, lethargy, diplopia (usually secondary to a sixth nerve palsy), transient visual obscurations, and papilledema. As intracranial pressure continues to rise, there may be bradycardia (50–60 beats/min), elevation of blood pressure, increase in systolic pressure associated with lowering or slight elevation of diastolic pressure, and a slowing of the respiratory rate. This is termed the Cushing reflex; it cannot be depended upon for the diagnosis of raised intracranial pressure.

AGENTS USED IN TREATING INTRACRANIAL PRESSURE

Hyperventilation

Hyperventilation may be used in acute situations (e.g., head trauma) and is often employed during neurosurgical procedures. Lowering the pCO_2 to 25–30 mm Hg causes vasoconstriction, reduced cerebral blood flow, an immediate reduction in intracerebral blood volume, and thus a decrease of intracranial pressure. Lowering pCO_2 below 25 mm Hg may be harmful because it reduces cerebral blood flow. If a patient brought to the emergency ward has rapid neurologic deterioration from increased intracranial pressure, whether due to trauma or to other intracranial processes, intubation and hyperventilation will often lower the pressure until such agents as mannitol take effect and specific neurosurgical treatment is instituted.

Mannitol

Mannitol, an osmotic dehydrating agent, is given 1–2 gm per kg
IV over 5–10 minutes, then 50–300 mg/kg IV every 6 hours,
depending on serum osmolarity. Onset of action is 15–30 minutes. It draws intracerebral water into the intravascular space
because of its hypertonicity and, for the same reason, induces
diuresis. It is usually not given for more than 24–48 hours and is
used in acute situations to "buy time" (e.g., after head trauma,
deterioration from an expanding intracranial process), often
prior to neurosurgical intervention. *Urea* is similar to mannitol
in its use, mode of action, and dose. These agents must be given
with caution to patients with renal and cardiac disease. There
may be "rebound" after their use (viz., return of water intracerebrally) because small amounts cross the blood-brain barrier.
Lower doses of mannitol (250 mg/kg) reduce the rebound
brain edema sometimes seen with mannitol. Diuretics such as
furosemide (Lasix) are often given as a supplement to mannitol.

Steroids

Steroids (dexamethasone) are used both acutely and chronically
(10 mg IV as initial dose, then 4–6 mg IV, IM, or orally every 6
hours). The onset of action is about 12 hours. Dexamethasone
is given in acute situations and may become the mainstay of
treatment after 12–24 hours. It is used palliatively to treat the
vasogenic edema associated with brain tumor, after some neurosurgical procedures, and often concomitantly with radiation
therapy to the brain. The mechanism of steroid action in these
situations is poorly understood. All patients receiving steroids
for more than a few hours should receive cimetidine or raniti-
dine and oral antacids. Steroids are probably not beneficial in
treating adults with trauma-induced cerebral edema or for cytotoxic edema associated with hypoxia, cerebral infarcts, or cerebral hemorrhage.

Glycerol

Glycerol, an osmotic dehydrating agent, is given orally or via
nasogastric tube in a dose of 1 gm/kg every 6 hours. It is slower

acting than mannitol/urea (onset of action is approximately 12 hours) but has the advantage that it can be used for longer periods and can be given orally. It does not have the side effects of prolonged steroid administration, and there is little "rebound." Although used infrequently, it may be used to treat swelling associated with cerebrovascular accidents, after neurosurgical procedures, or concomitantly with steroids.

Ventricular Puncture

Ventricular puncture may be done by a neurosurgeon when acute hydrocephalus occurs and mechanical release of raised intracranial pressure is needed. Causes include posterior fossa mass lesions, meningitis, and subarachnoid hemorrhage. Ventricular puncture may be done in the emergency room or on the ward.

Barbiturates

A controversial contribution to intracranial pressure control is the use of barbiturates. They are usually used when other attempts to lower intracranial pressure have failed and should only be used in conjunction with an intraventricular pressure monitor in an intensive care unit. Pentobarbital is the most widely used agent. Its mechanism of action in reducing intracranial pressure is unknown.

TREATMENT

When *transtentorial herniation* is in progress (see below), mannitol should be given immediately and neurosurgical consultation obtained. This refers to trauma, abrupt changes intracerebrally secondary to a vascular event, or deterioration after lumbar puncture. Concomitantly with mannitol administration, dexamethasone and furosemide should be given. If clinically appropriate, intubation and hyperventilation are also indicated.

In the *stroke patient* with a component of cerebral swelling or intracerebral hemorrhage (demonstrated by midline shift on CT scan accompanying decreased level of consciousness), corticosteroids appear to be of no value. Cerebral swelling secondary to thrombosis or embolus is most pronounced approximately 48 hours after the event; intracerebral hemorrhage may raise the intracranial pressure acutely. Such measures as fluid restriction and keeping the patient's head elevated are helpful. Hyperventilation may be indicated. In some centers, small doses of mannitol (0.25 gm/kg) and intracranial pressure monitoring are used.

Patients with *brain tumors* (primary or secondary) are often treated with steroids after diagnosis, during radiation therapy, and sometimes on a chronic basis. Interestingly, raised intracranial pressure due to metastatic brain tumor tends to respond better to steroids than that due to primary brain tumor.

Continuous monitoring of increased intracranial pressure with pressure monitoring devices is now possible and may be very useful in certain patients with severe head injury or stroke. Either an intraventricular cannula or a subarachnoid bolt can be used to monitor pressure and aid in therapeutic decisions.

HERNIATION SYNDROMES

There are three clinical syndromes of transtentorial herniation. Two represent loss of neurologic function that begins in the cerebral hemispheres and progresses to involve upper then lower brainstem, with death the usual result. The third consists of upward herniation of posterior fossa structures; it can also be fatal.

A. Uncal (lateral) syndrome of herniation
   1. A unilaterally dilated pupil is the first sign secondary to a mass in the middle fossa pushing against the uncus and trapping the third nerve. A contralateral hemiplegia is usually present. Respiration and consciousness are unimpaired.
   2. Progressive pressure leads to increasing stupor, a more complete third nerve palsy, and sometimes an ipsilateral hemiplegia with bilateral Babinski responses. The ipsilateral hemiplegia is secondary to tentorial pressure against the opposite cerebral peduncle (Kernohan's notch). Respiration may be normal or of the central neurogenic hyperventilation pattern. There is often decerebrate posturing (arms extended at the side with inward turning, either spontaneously or when a noxious

stimulus is applied). Decorticate posturing (arms flexed at the elbow "pointing" to the cortex) is not usually seen with the uncal syndrome.

3. Further pressure leads to prominent brainstem dysfunction with dilatation of both pupils, loss of brainstem reflexes (e.g., absent doll's eyes, no response to ice-water calorics), ataxic respiratory patterns, and bilateral decerebrate rigidity. Treatment at this stage is rarely of benefit.

B. Central syndrome of herniation

1. Pressure is exerted centrally on the diencephalon, rather than laterally as occurs in the uncal syndrome. The first sign is a change in alertness or behavior. Respiration is usually normal and contains frequent sighs or yawns. There may be Cheyne-Stokes respirations. Brainstem function is intact, although pupils are small but reactive to light, and there may be roving eye movements. Bilateral hyperreflexia and Babinski responses and rigidity of the extremities are usual. With progression there is decorticate posturing.

2. Involvement of upper brainstem leads to dilatation of both pupils and impairment of oculocephalic and oculovestibular reflexes (i.e., absent or abnormal doll's eyes or caloric response). Central neurogenic hyperventilation often occurs, and decorticate posturing progresses to decerebrate posturing. There may be wide fluctuation in body temperature.

3. Further progression leads to loss of all brainstem function with ataxic breathing, then apnea and death.

C. Posterior fossa herniation syndrome

1. Posterior fossa lesions may cause damage both by direct compression of the brainstem and by upward herniation through the tentorial hiatus. Upward herniation from the posterior fossa obliterates the ambient cisterns and aqueduct, causing hydrocephalus with obtundation and/or coma.

2. Midbrain compression produces an upward gaze deficit, while involvement of pontine pathways may cause sixth nerve palsies, ocular bobbing, and other oculomotor signs. In addition, anisocoria (asymmetric pupils) may lead to midposition fixed pupils.

These syndromes can develop over hours or minutes, depending on the pathologic process. The uncal syndrome is typically seen secondary to space-occupying lesions, such as intracranial hemorrhage or subdural hematoma, or tumor; central herniation is seen with diffuse increased intracranial pressure, e.g., Reye's syndrome or acute hydrocephalus. The posterior syndrome occurs with posterior fossa mass lesions.

Suggested Readings

Allen R. Intracranial pressure: a review of clinical problems, measurement techniques and monitoring methods. J Med Eng Technol 1986;10:299.

Aucoin PJ, Kotilairen HR, Gantz NM, Davidson R, Kelly P, Stone B. Intracranial pressure monitors. Epidemiologic study of risk factors and infections. Am J Med 1986;80:369.

Corbett JJ, Thompson HS. The rational management of idiopathic intracranial hypertension. Arch Neurol 1989;46:1049–1051.

Heffner JE, Sahn SA. Controlled hyperventilation in patients with intracranial hypertension. Application and management. Arch Intern Med 1983;143:765.

Lehman LB. Intracranial pressure monitoring and treatment: A contemporary view. Ann Emerg Med 1990;19:295–303.

Lyons MK, Meyer FB. Cerebrospinal fluid physiology and the management of increased intracranial pressure. Mayo Clin Proc 1990;65:684–707.

Roberts PA, Pollacy M, Engles C, Pendelton B, Reynolds E, Stevens FA. Effect on intracranial pressure of furosemide combined with varying doses and administration rates of mannitol. J Neurosurg 1987;66:440.

Ropper AH, Kennedy SF. Neurological and neurosurgical intensive care. 2nd ed. Rockville, MD: Aspen, 1988.

Chapter 28

Head Trauma

Head injury is a dynamic process. The most important parameters to monitor are the patient's level of consciousness and mental status. Below are important guidelines in dealing with the patient with head trauma:

1. In *severe head trauma,* control of airway and intravenous line placement are first priorities. One should assume that the patient has a fractured cervical spine and avoid turning the head; obtain cervical spine films in addition to skull film. Search for accompanying traumatic injury to abdominal and thoracic organs. If a patient has head injury and shock, assume that they are unrelated.

2. All patients with head trauma require *neurologic examination,* which must include (*a*) careful documentation of the patient's level of consciousness and ability to carry out mental tasks; (*b*) a careful look at the tympanic membranes for evidence of basilar skull fracture (blood or CSF):

    Carefully evaluate mental status.

    (*c*) scalp examination for evidence of localized areas of trauma; (*d*) precise recording of pupillary size and reaction; (*e*) check for hemiparesis and presence or absence of up-going toes.

3. *Concussion* is defined as an immediate and transient loss of consciousness or other neurologic function following head injury. There may be amnesia for events that occurred before and after the head injury.

4. *Observation in the hospital* for 24–48 hours and *neurosurgical consultation* are appropriate for a patient with any focal

abnormalities on neurologic examination, unconsciousness, abnormal mental status, skull fracture, or head trauma that is believed to be significant despite a normal examination. The decision to hospitalize or send home a patient who has not been unconscious and who has a normal neurologic examination must be made after careful consideration of the severity of the trauma and of who will look after and monitor the patient at home.

5. One of the most feared complications of head injury is the development of an acute *subdural* or *epidural hematoma*, which then may cause herniation (see Chapter 26) and fatal brainstem compression. Clinically, this process manifests itself as headache, decreased level of consciousness, and, late in the course, a dilated pupil that is usually on the side of the hematoma, secondary to pressure on the third nerve. *Epidural hematoma* most commonly represents arterial bleeding secondary to tearing the middle meningeal artery on the undersurface of the temporal bone. The patient may steadily deteriorate following the trauma or experience a "lucid interval" only to deteriorate later. Most (although not all) patients will have a fracture over the groove of the middle meningeal artery. *Subdural hematoma* is secondary to venous or arterial bleeding and similarly has the potential for brainstem compression. Subdural and epidural hematomas are diagnosed by CT scan or MRI.

6. There is potential danger and no value in performing a lumbar puncture in the patient with acute head trauma.

7. Skull films are an important part of the evaluation of a patient with significant head trauma and may show such abnormalities as depressed fractures, linear fractures in the middle fossa or base of the skull, or an air fluid level in the ethmoid sinus. Skull films should not, however, be requested before a CT scan in a patient with severe injury and should not be obtained for all patients with minor injuries.

8. MRI is of value in detecting areas of contusion or small hemorrhage in head trauma victims in the subacute or chronic stage. MRI is more sensitive than a CT scan in detecting subacute or chronic subdural hematomas.

Suggested Readings

Alberico AM, Ward JD, Choi SC, Marmarou A, Young HF. Outcome after severe head injury. Relationship to mass lesions, diffuse injury, and ICP course in pediatric and adult patients. J Neurosurg 1987;67:648.

Clifton GL. Controversies in medical management of head injury. Clin Neurosurg 1988;34:604.

Dwan PS, Becker DP, Gade G, Cheung M. Future therapy of head injury. Clin Neurosurg 1988;34:604.

Lillehei KO, Hoff JT. Advances in the management of closed head injury. Ann Emerg Med 1985;14:789.

Mandel S. Minor head injury may not be 'minor'. Postgrad Med 1989;85:213–225.

Meyer WJ. Central nervous system function in critical care. Surg Clin North Am 1983;63:401.

Rosenwasser RH, Andrews DW, Jimenez DF. Penetrating craniocerebral trauma. Surg Clin North Am 1991;71:305–316.

Young B, Rapp RP, Norton JA, Hoack D, Tibbs PA, Bean JR. Early prediction of outcome in head-injured patients. J Neurosurg 1981;54:300.

Chapter 29

Lumbar Puncture

INDICATIONS

1. When CNS infection (meningitis, encephalitis) is suspected, one must examine the CSF. Exception: Lumbar puncture should not be performed if one suspects brain abscess or another significant space-occupying mass lesion.
2. An LP is performed to determine whether CNS bleeding has occurred—e.g., to diagnose subarachnoid hemorrhage when that diagnosis is strongly suspected and the CT scan is negative, or to rule out bleeding prior to anticoagulation if a CT scan is unavailable.
3. An LP is done when CSF chemistries have diagnostic value—e.g., gamma globulin in multiple sclerosis.
4. Lumbar puncture is needed for the study of *CSF dynamics*—e.g., when checking for spinal block (performance of Queckenstedt test) or normal pressure hydrocephalus (performance of Katzman infusion or radionucleotide cisternography).
5. For cytology when carcinomatous or lymphomatous meningitis is suspected.
6. *Therapeutically,* an LP may be done to inject methotrexate for CNS leukemia or amphotericin B for fungal meningitis; to remove fluid as treatment for benign raised intracranial pressure or for the headache of subarachnoid hemorrhage.

CONTRAINDICATIONS

1. Infection at the site of the lumbar puncture.
2. Severe thrombocytopenia or uncorrected bleeding disorder.

3. When a cerebral *mass lesion* is suspected, particularly in a patient with lateralized neurologic signs or a possible mass in the posterior fossa.

- *Brain abscesses* (usually seen in congenital heart disease with right-to-left shunts, otitis media, or lung disease) may produce transtentorial or foramen magnum herniation after LP.
- *Brain tumors* may lead to herniation after LP, especially when located in the posterior fossa.
- *Subdural hematoma* is not usually diagnosed by LP, and the removal of fluid may be harmful.
- *Intracranial hemorrhage* is best diagnosed by CT scan.

In these instances, a CT scan or MRI for definition of the midline and a search for a mass lesion should be done before the LP.

4. Lumbar puncture must not be done in the presence of *papilledema* (a check of the fundi must precede each LP). An LP may ultimately be done in a patient with papilledema (e.g., in pseudotumor or if CSF examination is crucial), but only after neurologic and/or neurosurgical consultation.

COMPLICATIONS

Post-LP headache occurs in 10–30% of patients. It is characteristically exacerbated by sitting or standing, and relieved by lying flat. It is seen within the first 1–3 days after the LP; it usually lasts 2–5 days, although it may persist for weeks. Treatment consists of bed rest and fluids. (The mechanism of the headache is believed to be continued CSF leakage through the dural hole at the site of the LP, with subsequent intracranial traction on the meninges.) Severe leaks can be treated by the placement of a blood patch by an anesthesiologist or neurosurgeon. Post-LP headache may be minimized by using a small-gauge needle (22 or 20), inserting the needle parallel to the dural fibers so they are spread apart rather than torn, and having the patient turn prone before removing the needle. Having the patient lie in bed post-LP may or may not be useful. Patients with migraine are particularly prone to post-LP headaches.

When there is an unexpected *raised opening pressure* (it must stay elevated after the patient has relaxed with legs extended and 10 minutes have elapsed from the onset of the LP), remove minimal fluid needed for studies. Neurologic and/or neurosurgical consultation should be obtained, the use of mannitol and/or steroids considered, and the patient watched carefully over the ensuing hours for signs of deterioration. Patients with meningitis may have markedly elevated pressures, but these pressures are not as dangerous as raised intracranial pressure secondary to a focal lesion. Remember, hypercarbia, water intoxication, and hypertensive encephalopathy are remediable causes of raised intracranial pressure. When the intracranial pressure is raised and there is neurologic deterioration immediately or during the hours after the LP, treatment with osmotic dehydrating agents and steroids is indicated (see Chapter 27).

If the patient has a partial or almost complete *spinal block* secondary to compression of the cord (e.g., by tumor) CSF removal may cause rapid worsening of the block. Signs of block include abnormal manometric findings and xanthochromic fluid (raised protein) under low pressure (see Chapter 14 for treatment).

METHOD

1. The puncture is carried out in the midline between the L3-L4 or L4-L5 interspaces located by the level of the iliac crest.
2. Insert the bevel of the needle parallel to the long axis of the spine.
3. If manometric studies and myelography are not being performed, use a 20- or 22-gauge needle.
4. Note the opening and closing pressures as well as the amount of fluid removed.
5. Coughing or abdominal pressure causes delayed venous return around the cord and should increase CSF flow and pressure. These maneuvers show that the needle is in place, but they do not test for spinal subarachnoid block. To do this, raise the jugular pressure (via hand pressure or a blood pressure cuff around the neck) and measure the rise and fall of CSF pressure. Manometric studies are not done routinely and are never performed if the baseline pressure is elevated or an intracranial lesion is suspected.
6. *Proper positioning* of the patient is crucial for successful lumbar puncture. The patient should be placed in the fetal

position with his back at right angles to the bed. Insert the needle under the skin (after local anesthesia) and then decide on the angle of entry. Make sure the needle is strictly parallel to the bed and angled toward the patient's umbilicus. Once the needle has been advanced, if it does not enter the subarachnoid space or if it encounters bone, the direction of the needle cannot be changed. Pull the needle back to just beneath the skin and redirect it. With experience, one will learn to recognize the familiar "pop" as the needle enters the subarachnoid space. If the LP is not possible in the fetal position, have patient sit up and lean forward grasping a pillow; try again in the sitting position (it is easier to gauge the midline). Remember, pressure measurements are difficult to interpret in the sitting position, and it may be useful to have the patient lie down after the needle is inserted.

7. When an LP is impossible because of bony anomalies or local infection, and CSF examination is crucial, one should arrange for a cisternal or cervical (C1-C2) tap under fluoroscopy.

EXAMINATION OF THE CSF

1. *Collect four tubes* of fluid: One tube is used for cell count, one for chemistries, and a third for bacteriologic studies. One tube is saved for future use, e.g., a sample may be lost, an unexpected chemistry value may require a repeat determination, or a new test may be wanted. If a traumatic tap is suspected, cells are counted in both the first and fourth tubes. Some send tubes 1 and 4 for cell count with 1 ml in each, tubes 2 and 3 for chemistries and bacteriology. To determine whether a "traumatic tap" has occurred, fluid can be spun in a centrifuge and the presence of xanthochromia noted. A repeat tap is done at a higher interspace.

2. If red blood cells (RBCs) are present, count them in the first and third tubes. In subarachnoid or intracranial bleeding, the amount of blood remains constant in each tube, and the blood does not clot. Decreasing numbers of cells suggest a traumatic tap. After centrifugation, the CSF from a traumatic tap will be clear, while with true CNS bleeding

the supernatant is xanthochromic if the bleeding occurred at least 2 to 4 hours previously. Finding crenated RBCs is of no distinguishing value, since they appear both with true bleeding and after traumatic taps.

3. Check to see if the CSF is *clear* by comparing it with water. A CSF protein level greater than 100 mg/10 ml usually causes the spinal fluid to look faintly yellow. Approximately 200–300 white blood cells (WBCs) are needed to cause CSF cloudiness. Dark CSF may be seen with metastatic melanoma and jaundice with hyperbilirubinemia; subdural hematoma may produce xanthochromia.

4. Always examine the CSF for *cells* within 1 hour after LP and preferably sooner. Normally, there should be no polymorphonuclear neutrophils (PMNs) and no more than five mononuclear cells. It is very important to distinguish between RBCs and WBCs. After a total cell count is done, add acetic acid to the spinal fluid; this lyses the RBCs but leaves the WBCs intact. (Rinse a capillary tube with acetic acid and then draw the CSF into the tube.) Often one can distinguish between PMNs and lymphocytes by adding methylene blue to the fluid. When looking for tumor cells, or if the nature of the WBCs in the CSF is questioned, a Millipore, cytocentrifuge, or cytologic examination is indicated. When bacterial or tuberculous infection is suspected, perform a Gram stain and an acid-fast stain on the centrifuged sediment. When fungal disease is a possibility, do an India ink preparation. (Place a coverslip over one drop of CSF on a slide. Place a drop of India ink next to the coverslip and allow it to seep under. Check at the interface for *Cryptococcus*.)

5. When there are RBCs in the CSF and the patient has a normal complete blood count, expect approximately one WBC for every 700 RBCs (make further corrections for anemia). In addition, every 700 RBCs raise the protein by 1 mg/100 ml.

INTERPRETATION

Glucose

Increased glucose levels are usually not significant, merely reflecting systemic hyperglycemia. With changing blood glucose, CSF glucose lags blood glucose by approximately 1 hour, and the level is approximately two-thirds that of blood glucose. In the face of systemic hyperglycemia, a concomitant blood glucose determination is needed to demonstrate a relatively lowered CSF glucose (e.g., suggesting infection) that might otherwise be considered normal.

Decreased glucose levels are seen in bacterial, tuberculous, and fungal meningitis, and sometimes with meningeal involvement by neoplasm or a nontuberculous granulomatous process, such as sarcoidosis. Although characteristically normal in viral infections, the CSF glucose level has been reported to be low with certain CNS viral infections (herpes, mumps, lymphocytic choriomeningitis). Decreased CSF glucose is secondary to changes in carbohydrate metabolism by neural tissue, WBC use of glucose, and alteration of glucose transport into the CNS.

Protein

Protein levels are increased in a wide variety of neurologic diseases and usually reflect an abnormality in the blood-brain barrier. Elevated levels are seen in processes affecting nerve roots in peripheral neuropathy. Normal CSF protein is less than 45 mg/100 ml. Common processes producing increased CSF protein are as follows:

1. *Diabetes* frequently causes protein elevations (up to 150 mg/100 ml, or even higher when significant peripheral neuropathy is present). Look for unrecognized diabetes when there is an unexpected protein elevation. The mechanism is probably related to dorsal root ganglia involvement.
2. *Brain tumor* frequently produces protein elevations of 100–200 mg/100 ml, although the level may be normal. Marked increases are seen in meningiomas, acoustic neuromas, and tumors near the ventricles, e.g., ependymomas. CSF protein in brainstem gliomas is generally normal. Encapsulated *brain abscesses* produce elevations similar to those seen in brain tumors.
3. *Spinal cord tumors* also raise protein levels, often to extremely high levels (e.g., 750–1000 mg/100 ml), especially when block is present.

4. *Multiple sclerosis* may cause protein elevation in some patients, but the elevation is usually mild. Protein levels greater than 80 mg/100 ml in a patient with multiple sclerosis make the diagnosis suspect.

5. *Acute purulent meningitis* invariably elevates the protein level regardless of the cause, as do subacute and chronic granulomatous meningitis. Viral infections of the CNS are associated with normal protein levels or mild increases in protein initially with a rise later, which serves as a clue to the diagnosis. Carcinomatous meningitis causes significant elevation of CSF protein.

6. *Infectious polyneuritis* (Guillain-Barré syndrome) characteristically causes increased protein levels. The protein is frequently normal during the first few days of the illness but rises after 1 week.

7. *Syphilis* produces increased protein levels in the meningovascular form and general paresis; the CSF may be normal in long-standing tabes.

8. Mild to moderate elevations may be seen in myxedema, uremia, connective tissue disorders, and Cushing's disease.

9. *Cerebrovascular disease* generally causes no protein elevation or only mild increases. There may however, be large increases with cerebral hemorrhage because of serum protein in the CSF.

Gamma Globulin

The measurement of gamma globulin is used most frequently to support the diagnosis of multiple sclerosis. Normally, gamma globulin represents 13–15% or less of total protein. (If total protein values are less than 20 mg/100 ml, the percentage of gamma globulin may be quite unreliable.) Gamma globulin is elevated in multiple sclerosis, subacute sclerosing panencephalitis, general paresis, herpes encephalitis, myxedema, some cases of carcinomatous cerebellar degeneration, and some connective tissue diseases. Measurement of IgG:albumin ratio (normally less than 0.18), measurement of IgG synthesis rate, or detection of oligoclonal bands provides similar information.

CSF Pressure

The *CSF pressure* is normally less than 200 mm H_2O with the patient lying down (or at the level of the foramen magnum in the sitting position). It is not affected by changes in systemic blood pressure but is exquisitely sensitive to changes in blood CO_2 (hyperventilation lowers intracranial pressure) and venous pressure.

1. Elevated pressures are seen in acute bacterial, fungal, and viral meningitis and in meningoencephalitis.
2. Pressure elevation is frequent with tumors or other intra-cerebral mass lesions (e.g., abscess), although pressure may be normal despite a large tumor.
3. Pressure is usually elevated in intracerebral bleeding and in subarachnoid hemorrhage.
4. Interestingly, the pressure and protein may be raised, and there may be papilledema with polyneuritis or spinal tumor.
5. Unexplained elevated pressures may be due to congestive heart failure, chronic obstructive pulmonary disease, hyper-capnia, jugular venous obstruction, or pericardial effusion.
6. *Pseudotumor cerebri* (benign raised intracranial pressure) refers to raised pressure, as high as 400–600 mm H_2O, with papilledema, not associated with a mass lesion or hydro-cephalus, and with an otherwise normal CSF. Causes include withdrawal from steroids, pregnancy and menarche, hypo-or hypervitaminosis A, hyperparathyroidism, tetracycline or phenothiazine administration, and venous sinus occlusion. Female patients with pseudotumor are frequently obese. Often the cause is unknown. One must first rule out tumor and hydrocephalus (usually with CT scan or MRI) and then establish the diagnosis with LP. Lumbar punctures alone are sometimes sufficient to lower CSF pressure and reverse the process. Acetazolamide may be given to decrease CSF pro-duction, and then steroids are administered if necessary. Transient visual disturbances, such as blurring and dim-ming, are common in pseudotumor. More severe visual diffi-culties, such as field defects and actual loss of vision, can also occur and warrant vigorous treatment of the increased pressure, including lumbar peritoneal shunts and surgical decompression in protracted cases. Frequent monitoring of visual fields and of the optic nerve is therefore warranted.

Pleocytosis

PMNs in the CSF suggest a bacterial infection, and lymphocytes suggest a viral or chronic inflammatory process (although PMNs are sometimes seen at the onset of a viral infection). WBCs may be seen after subarachnoid hemorrhage, thrombosis, and, at times, with infectious mononucleosis. Eosinophils suggest a parasitic infection or dye reaction. Remember, many organic diseases of the CNS produce a mild pleocytosis. A thorough bacteriologic investigation must be carried out in all instances, even though cells do not always represent infection. Carcinomatous meningitis tends to be accompanied by fewer than 100 cells in the CSF (more than 100 cells suggests an infectious process). T cell and B cell markers should be checked if the WBC count in the CSF is elevated and lymphomatous meningitis is suspected. The initial tap may be negative for tumor cells. The yield is increased on repeated cytologic examinations. (Red cells are discussed in Chapter 5.)

NOTE: If upon CSF analysis the cell count, protein, and glucose are all normal, it is highly unlikely that additional studies on the spinal fluid will be useful (unless special considerations exist—e.g., gamma globulin determination in suspected multiple sclerosis).

Suggested Readings

Ahlskog J, O'Neill B. Pseudotumor cerebri. Ann Intern Med 1982;97:249.

Fishman RA. Cerebrospinal fluid in diseases of the nervous system. Philadelphia: WB Saunders, 1980.

Gorelick PB, Biller J. Lumbar puncture. Technique, indications and complications. Postgrad Med 1986;79:257.

Marton KI, Geon AD. The spinal tap: a new look at an old test. Ann Intern Med 1986;104:840.

Hayward RA, Shapiro MF. Laboratory testing on cerebrospinal fluid: a reappraisal. Lancet 1987;1:1.

Pearce JMS. Hazards of lumbar puncture. Br Med J 1982;285:1521.

Chapter 30

Neurodiagnostic Procedures

ELECTROENCEPHALOGRAM (EEG)

The EEG is a physiologic monitor of cerebral cortical function. It measures electrical activity that is generated in the cerebral cortex and then synchronized and modulated by thalamic and reticular activating structures. It is primarily a measure of gray matter or neuronal function and is abnormal when there is disease impinging on neurons or gray matter. The EEG is usually not abnormal in white matter disease.

1. *Seizure disorders.* The EEG is a central test for the diagnosis and management of patients with seizure disorders. It should be emphasized that not all patients with clinically definite seizure disorders have abnormalities on EEG, and conversely, paroxysmal EEG abnormalities are sometimes seen in people without seizure disorders. During an actual seizure, an EEG usually demonstrates massive electrical discharge, followed in the postictal period by slowing. Interictal EEGs in patients with seizure disorders are abnormal in approximately 70% of patients. Certain seizure disorders are classified according to EEG patterns:

   a. *Absence,* a seizure characterized by brief losses of consciousness (e.g., staring spells of no more than several seconds), occurs almost exclusively between the ages of 5 and 18. It shows classic 3 per second spike and wave discharges. The diagnosis of petit mal depends on this EEG finding.

b. *Temporal lobe epilepsy* is characterized by focal EEG abnormalities in either or both temporal lobes, including sharp waves or spike discharges. These abnormalities may not be apparent on routine interictal EEGs but can usually be demonstrated by sleep EEGs, nasopharyngeal or sphenoidal leads, or special scalp leads over the temporal regions. If temporal lobe epilepsy is suspected, such procedures should be carried out, and continuous monitoring may be necessary in difficult cases.

The administration of anticonvulsants does not necessarily affect the EEG, although certain medications cause specific EEG patterns (e.g., barbiturates and benzodiazepines cause beta or fast wave patterns). Patients with a seizure disorder who remain seizure free for 2 years and have an EEG that reverts to normal can usually be weaned off medication with a high likelihood of success. In treating people with seizure disorders, it is very important to remember that one must "treat the patient" and not the EEG.

2. *Cerebrovascular disease.* The EEG can be useful in differentiating cortical from subcortical strokes. In general, patients with involvement of cortex secondary to large vessel disease usually have abnormalities on EEG, while small vessel subcortical or brainstem infarctions are associated with normal EEG patterns. The EEG may clarify a clinical suspicion of stroke when the initial CT scan is normal early in the course. New onset of seizures in old age is often a clinical clue for unsuspected cerebrovascular disease.

3. *Metabolic encephalopathy.* Patients with metabolic encephalopathy of any cause have abnormal EEGs, consisting of nonfocal slowing of the EEG pattern or rhythmic bursts of symmetrical frontal slowing. The EEG can be useful in identifying metabolic encephalopathies or in ruling out metabolic encephalopathies in patients with altered mental status. Sometimes these patterns can be quite helpful, e.g., the "triphasic" waves of hepatic encephalopathy.

4. *Tumors.* Depending on the location and size of a tumor, the EEG is often abnormal, with either focal slowing or spike

discharges. New onset of seizures in middle age is often the presenting symptom of tumor. However, the CT scan or MRI is the major test used to diagnose tumors or other space-occupying lesions.

5. *Other diseases.* Some disorders have characteristic EEG findings (e.g., Jakob-Creutzfeldt disease, herpes simplex encephalitis, SSPE). Some infectious disorders of the central nervous system do not affect the brain wave (e.g., cryptococcal meningitis). Psychiatric diseases (affective disorders, schizophrenia) usually have no effect on the EEG. Migraine headaches may be associated with focal slowing. Posttraumatic contusions may cause focal slowing or even paroxysmal activity. The EEG is often used as an adjunct in the diagnosis of brain death.

NOTE: Ambulatory EEG monitoring (analogous to Holter ECG) may be useful in detecting paroxysmal abnormalities, such as seizure discharges, not seen on individual EEG recordings.

ELECTROMYOGRAPHY

The electromyogram is an electrical test measuring physiologic function in muscle. It is used to help diagnose muscle disease, disease of the neuromuscular junction, and denervation of muscles secondary to nerve or root lesions.

1. *Myopathy.* Patients with myopathy often show certain features: (a) low-amplitude, short-duration motor unit potentials; (b) complex polyphasic motor unit potentials; (c) increased insertional activity (e.g., bizarre high frequency discharges). It is usually not possible to distinguish one myopathy from another by EMG. Some myopathies (e.g., polymyositis and muscular dystrophies) may show fibrillation potentials.

2. *Myotonia* presents a characteristic pattern of hyperexcitability with persistent waxing and waning and repetitive discharges, which sound myographically like a "dive bomber." The dive bomber pattern is not diagnostic of any single myotonic disorder but is characteristic of myotonia.

3. *Neuromuscular junction (NMJ) disorders.* Presynaptic NMJ disorders (e.g., botulism, Eaton-Lambert syndrome) may be characterized by progressive enhancement of motor unit action potentials evoked by repetitive stimulation of the motor nerve. Most also show normal amplitude miniature endplate potentials. By contrast, postsynaptic NMJ disorders (e.g., myasthenia gravis) show a decremental response of the muscle action potential with repetitive nerve stimulation and subnormal amplitudes of the miniature endplate potentials. Both pre- and postsynaptic EMGs show increased jitter or variation in latency between a nerve stimulus and the resulting muscle action potentials on single fiber EMG testing.

4. *Denervation* produces increased polyphasic action potentials, bizarre high-frequency discharges, fibrillations, positive sharp waves, and fasciculations. Fibrillation potentials develop 3–4 weeks after the onset of nerve injury. Thus, someone with an acute root or nerve lesion may not show muscle fibrillation. Examination of muscle groups in the legs or arms may help to diagnose specific root lesions and whether denervated muscles are referable to a single root. Similarly, denervation can be used to help diagnose amyotrophic lateral sclerosis or other anterior horn cell diseases. Disorders of the proximal nerve, including the cell body, will prolong the "F response," which is a peripherally recorded potential produced by retrograde conduction of a stimulated action potential to the soma, with subsequent orthograde conduction back to the periphery. The Hoffman, or H, reflex is an orthograde motor potential generated by stimulating sensory fibers in the stretch reflex arc. Thus, an H reflex can be used to detect either sensory or motor root lesions. The "F response" is particularly useful in disorders that primarily affect the proximal nerve (e.g., early stages of Guillain-Barré syndrome).

NERVE CONDUCTION VELOCITIES

Nerve conduction velocities yield information pertaining to the integrity of both myelin and axon in peripheral nerve. If nerve conduction velocity is slowed in all limbs, a *generalized* neuropathy is implied (e.g., diabetic or alcoholic neuropathies).

Disorders that primarily affect myelin (e.g., Guillain-Barré) cause nerve conduction slowing out of proportion to EMG changes, while "axonal" neuropathies (e.g., due to alcohol) cause EMG changes of denervation out of proportion to nerve conduction abnormalities. Individual nerve abnormalities can be seen in nerve entrapments (e.g., carpal tunnel) or nerve infarction or damage (e.g., mononeuritis multiplex).

EVOKED POTENTIALS

An evoked potential is an electrical response recorded from the central nervous system, elicited by an external stimulus—visual, auditory, or somatosensory. Evoked potentials are useful in localizing subtle sensory lesions and in detecting unsuspected *subclinical* sensory deficits.

1. *Visual evoked responses* (VERs), measured over the occiput, are stimulated by shifting checkerboard patterns in the visual fields. They are most helpful in demonstrating lesions in the optic nerves and are particularly useful in diagnosis of multiple sclerosis. Most patients with a history of optic neuritis or multiple sclerosis have VER abnormalities. VER changes are also seen in toxic and nutritional amblyopias, tumors compressing the anterior visual pathways, Friedreich's ataxia, and pernicious anemia. VERs may also be of benefit in patients suspected of hysterical visual loss. They are helpful in monitoring optic nerve and chiasm function in patients with pituitary tumors or pseudotumor cerebri.

2. *Brainstem auditory evoked responses* (BAERs) are elicited by delivering click stimuli to either ear. Their major advantage is the ability to localize auditory pathway lesions to eighth nerve, cochlear nucleus, superior olive, lateral lemniscus, or inferior colliculus. They are exquisitely sensitive to extrinsic lesions, such as acoustic neuromas, and may detect these lesions before they are visible by CT scan. They are also sensitive to intrinsic brainstem lesions involving the auditory pathways as seen in multiple sclerosis, brainstem glioma, brainstem infarcts, and olivopontocerebellar degeneration. Because they are not abolished by high doses of anesthesia or barbiturates, they are useful monitors of brainstem integrity in patients rendered comatose or treated with

these agents. They may prove useful as prognostic indicators in the comatose patient, especially after head trauma.

3. *Somatosensory evoked responses* (SERs) are elicited by stimulating large fiber sensory systems peripherally. Tibial and peroneal evoked responses may help to localize lesions to their respective peripheral nerves, lumbosacral plexus, dorsal spinal cord, spinomedullary junction, brainstem, and thalamus. Median nerve SERs will assess function across Erb's point, and centrally through spinomedullary junction, brainstem, and thalamus. Pudendal SERs help to detect deficits of sensory innervation of the genitalia. Virtually any lesion compromising conduction in these systems (e.g., multiple sclerosis, spinal cord tumors, severe cervical spondylosis) may produce SER abnormalities. SERs are useful adjuncts to monitor spinal cord function during cord surgery.

MAGNETIC RESONANCE IMAGING (MRI)

Magnetic resonance imaging is rapidly becoming the imaging modality of choice for a variety of neurologic disorders, including congenital anomalies, especially those involving the posterior fossa (e.g., Arnold-Chiari); pathology of the sella turcica, including pituitary tumors; lesions involving the internal auditory canal (e.g., acoustic neuroma); lesions of the posterior fossa, including brainstem and cerebellum (e.g., brainstem gliomas, cerebellar astrocytoma), lesions of temporal lobes and white matter diseases, especially those of demyelinating origin (e.g., multiple sclerosis); spinal cord lesion (e.g., spinal cord tumors, syringomyelia).

An MRI scan takes approximately 30–60 minutes, and during most of this time, the patient must lie motionless. If this is not possible, sedation may be required. A scan consists of pulsating radio waves (heard as clicking sounds by the patient) and the magnetic field (which the patient does not feel). An important note to the house officer is that t*he magnetic field is always on.* Severe harm can occur to a patient if someone enters the scan room with a metallic object (such as a stethoscope, tuning fork, reflex hammer, etc.). An MRI cannot be performed in patients with pacemakers, intracranial aneurysm clips, or a metallic foreign body in the eye or brain.

The areas of the nervous system where MRI has a particular advantage over CT are those where there is significant bony artifact (especially brainstem and spinal cord). MRI continues to have limitations when there is poor patient cooperation and movement precludes a prolonged period with the patient still; or when the issue is deciding whether acute hemorrhage has occurred—e.g. subarachnoid hemorrhage. Advances in software and in altering pulse sequences may resolve these problems in the future.

Points of particular interest with respect to MRI imaging of the nervous system include the following:

1. *Neuroanatomy.* MRI provides a unique opportunity to visualize the neuroanatomy involved in normal and abnormal function of the nervous system. Thus, the components of the pyramidal and extrapyramidal motor system, the sensory system of the face and body, and the visual, hearing, and olfactory systems can be easily visualized in three planes. House officers and students are urged to use MRI as a valuable tool to enhance their knowledge of functional neuroanatomy and to identify the lesions and structures involved in the disease processes encountered.

2. *Degenerative brain diseases.* MRI may be helpful in visualizing and in better understanding certain degenerative diseases. For example, it appears that the deposition of iron is increased in the putamen in Parkinson's disease and varies from the pattern in other basal ganglia degenerations.

3. *Seizures.* MRI has become the imaging modality of choice in the evaluation of patients with new-onset seizures. Reasons for its superiority over CT in this clinical problem include:

   a. Its ability to image in three planes makes it more sensitive in detecting lesions that may cause seizures and in delineating their size and location. The coronal views are particularly valuable in detecting temporal lobe lesions.

   b. Seizures may be caused by arteriovenous malformations (AVMs), which are imaged very well by MRI without the necessity for intravenous contrast injection.

   c. Neoplasms, either primary or secondary, may be responsible for seizures, and MRI is extremely sensitive for detecting the presence of tumors. Edema surrounding tumor is well seen with MRI.

4. *Headaches.* MRI is proving particularly valuable in the evaluation of patients with chronic headaches because of its ability to detect brain tumor, AVM, cerebral venous thrombosis, subdural hematomas, aneurysms, or hydrocephalus.

5. *Stroke.* CT remains the imaging modality of choice in the setting of acute stroke to exclude the presence of hemorrhage. MRI is more sensitive (*a*) in the subacute stage to detect subtle hemorrhage; (*b*) in imaging infarct, especially within the first 48 hours after symptom onset; (*c*) in detecting infarcts in the posterior fossa; (*d*) in detecting other lesions masquerading as stroke, such as brain tumor; and (*e*) in detecting cavernous sinus thrombosis.

6. *Head trauma.* CT remains the appropriate study in the acute evaluation of the trauma patient, in searching for an extraaxial blood clot or assessing acute brain damage. MRI is preferred in the subacute state to detect extra axial hematoma, contusion, and shearing injury.

7. *Ataxia/deafness/vertigo.* MRI is preferred over CT in evaluating the posterior fossa since, unlike with CT scanning, there are no bony artifacts. It is particularly valuable in imaging cerebellar neoplasms (astrocytoma, medulloblastoma), neoplasms of the brainstem, and acoustic neuromas or other lesions in the cerebellopontine angle (CPA).

8. *Dementia.* MRI is quite valuable in evaluation of the patient with dementia, because of its ability to detect and delineate tumors, subdural hematoma, multiinfarcts, and cerebral atrophy (see Chapter 10).

9. *Multiple sclerosis.* MRI is superior to CT in detecting the demyelinating lesions of multiple sclerosis. Patients without clinical evidence of brain involvement (e.g., when presenting with optic neuritis or a spinal cord lesion) are frequently found to have characteristic periventricular lesions on MRI.

10. *Spine and spinal cord.* MRI is becoming the imaging examination of choice for disorders that affect the spine or spinal cord. It is of particular value for visualizing primary spinal cord tumors (e.g., gliomas), intradural or extradural processes that impinge on the spinal cord (e.g., meningiomas, metastatic tumors), syringomyelia, hematomyelia,

and spinal stenosis. Its role in relation to CT and myelography in evaluating cervical and lumbar disc disease is still being defined, but it is already playing a major role in evaluating these processes. The interested reader is referred to the excellent review by Hyman and Gorey.

11. *Visual loss.* MRI has demonstrated its value in imaging lesions in the orbit such as optic glioma or when due to a mass lesion compressing the optic chiasm.

12. *Amenorrhea/galactorrhea.* These symptoms may be due to a pituitary microadenoma. Currently, the sensitivity of MRI in detecting pituitary microadenomas is equal to or greater than contrast-enhanced direct coronal thin-section CT. MRI is superior in delineating invasion of local structures (e.g., cavernous sinus) by macroadenomas.

13. *Congenital anomalies.* MRI is an excellent modality to demonstrate congenital anomalies, such as Dandy-Walker cyst in the posterior fossa, Arnold-Chiari malformation, and agenesis of the corpus callosum. It provides details of abnormal morphology in the dysmorphic brain—e.g. in derangements of myelination.

The recent introduction of paramagnetic contrast media as an adjunct to magnetic resonance imaging will no doubt further enhance the value of MRI and likely make it the procedure of choice in even more clinical situations than at present. Those situations include searching for brain and leptomeningeal metastases.

CT SCAN

Computerized axial tomography heralded a revolution in the diagnosis and management of neurologic disease. Its use has lessened considerably with the development of MRI.

Use of contrast in CT scanning. CT scans need not necessarily be done with contrast enhancement, and that decision should depend on the clinical situation. Contrast enhancement is generally used to assist diagnosis of certain infections and tumors. The danger of "routine" contrast use relates to allergy to the dye and the effect of dye on renal function.

1. *Cerebrovascular disease.* The basic value of the CT scan in

cerebrovascular disease is to differentiate hemorrhage from infarction. Virtually all hemorrhages show up as increased density on CT scans, while either no abnormality or decreased density is seen with infarction. This distinction is particularly important when it is impossible to distinguish infarction from hemorrhage on clinical grounds alone, since treatment is drastically different with these two conditions. *No* patient should be anticoagulated without prior CT scan to rule out bleeding. Lumbar puncture is less sensitive than CT scan in identifying intracranial hemorrhage. Fifteen to 20% of infarcts are apparent immediately on CT scan, and most moderate-sized infarcts are apparent at 3–5 days. The diagnosis of multiple infarcts due to emboli can also be made by CT scan, including infarcts seen in areas that have not declared themselves clinically. CT scan can identify arteriovenous malformations and aneurysms, although the precise diagnosis of these disorders usually requires arteriography.

2. *Tumors.* Virtually all tumors larger than 2–4 mm can be seen on CT scan. Depending on the pattern, certain diagnostic interpretations can be made. CT scan sensitivity to tumors is enhanced by perfusion with iodinated contrast agents.

3. *Hydrocephalus.* The CT scan and MRI have replaced pneumoencephalography for the demonstration and evaluation of hydrocephalus.

4. *Degenerative disease.* Patients with CNS degenerative diseases, such as Alzheimer's disease, usually have abnormal CT scans. However, as patients get older, they usually have widened sulci and enlarged ventricles due to loss of brain tissue. Increase in depth of sulci does not necessarily correlate with dementia and can also be seen in "normal" people. There are patients with degenerative disease or dementia who have normal-appearing CT scans.

5. *Demyelinating disease.* In a small percentage of patients with demyelinating disease, abnormalities may be seen on CT scan. Periventricular white matter lesions may be visualized, especially if carried out with contrast. MRI is more sensitive for these lesions.

6. *Subdural hematoma.* Approximately 80% of subdural hematomas, both unilateral and bilateral, can be seen on

CT scan. Some subdurals may be isodense and not visualized by CT scan; they require arteriography or brain scanning for diagnosis.

7. *Brainstem and spinal cord.* In general, the brainstem and spinal cord are better visualized on MRI than CT scan. Disease of neural foramina—e.g., disc and bony disease—are better evaluated by CT than by MRI. CT scanning is limited by the fact that one cannot image the entire spinal cord in horizontal sections. Thus, spinal CT scans should be reserved for clinical situations in which the examination suggests abnormality at a specific spinal level.

8. *Trauma.* CT is effective in differentiating a wide variety of consequences of trauma in the nervous system, including fractures, epidural and subdural hematomas, and shifts of intracranial contents. CT scanning is an excellent screening method for showing intracranial shifts prior to performing lumbar puncture.

ARTERIOGRAPHY

Cerebral arteriography is used to define vascular disease of both intracranial and extracranial vessels, e.g., carotid artery disease, arteriovenous malformation, and aneurysms. Digital arterial angiography allows computer-enhanced views of the carotid arteries without the risk of arteriography but is being used less to evaluate carotid disease. Magnetic resonance angiography (MRA) is being developed rapidly at many centers and may replace conventional angiography in the future. (See Chapter 5.)

Suggested Readings

Brant-Zawadzki M, Norman D. Magnetic resonance imaging of the central nervous system. New York: Raven, 1987.

Chiappa KH, Ropper AH. Evoked potentials in clinical medicine. N Engl J Med 1982;306:1140,1205.

Gilmore R. Evoked potentials. Neurol Clin 1988;6(4).

Goodgold J, Eberstein A. Electrodiagnosis of neuromuscular diseases. 3rd ed. Baltimore: Williams & Wilkins, 1983.

Hyman RA, Gorey MT. Imaging strategies for MR of the brain. Radiol Clin North Am 1988;26:471.

Johnson E. Practical electromyography. Baltimore: Williams & Wilkins, 1980.

Niedermeyer E, daSilva F. Electroencephalopathy. 2nd ed. Baltimore: Urban & Schwarzenberg, 1987.

Stark DD, Bradley WG. Magnetic resonance imaging. St. Louis: CV Mosby, 1988.

Spehlman R. Evoked potential primer. Boston: Butterworth, 1985.

Chapter 31

Neuroanatomy

A *destructive lesion* in the hemisphere or subcortex causes eyes to deviate toward the same side as the lesion. Thus, with a right-sided lesion the eyes are deviated to the right. An *excitatory lesion* at the cortical level (viz., a seizure) causes eyes to deviate to the contralateral side. Thus, with a left-sided seizure, eyes are deviated to the right. A *destructive lesion* in the pons (after fibers have crossed) causes eyes to deviate to the side opposite the damage. Thus, with a left-sided lesion, eyes deviate to the right. (There are no excitatory lesions of the pons.) Eye deviation secondary to hemisphere lesions, but not brainstem lesions, may be overcome by brainstem reflexes, e.g., doll's eyes maneuver.

1. *Blindness in one eye* represents retinal or optic nerve dysfunction. The optic nerve is frequently involved in multiple sclerosis (optic neuritis), producing unilateral blindness; it may also be involved by tumor (optic glioma) or undergo atrophy secondary to prolonged raised intracranial pressure. The optic nerve may also be affected by vascular processes such as giant cell arteritis and amaurosis fugax.
2. *Bitemporal hemianopsia* is classically found in the pituitary tumors secondary to pressure on the optic chiasm. Nonhomonymous field defects usually imply a chiasmal lesion. Remember, concentric tunnel vision may be seen in hysterical blindness.
3. *Homonymous hemianopsia* implies a lesion posterior to the chiasm. It may involve optic tract or optic radiations emanating from the lateral geniculate body (or the lateral geniculate itself). The closer a lesion is to the lateral geniculate, the

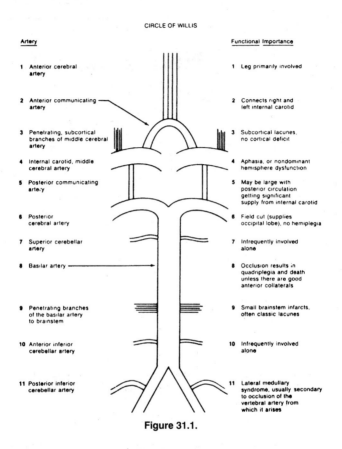

Figure 31.1.

smaller it can be and still produce a homonymous hemianopsia. Occlusions of the posterior cerebral artery usually produce homonymous hemianopsia with sparing of the macula.

4. The *optic radiations* fan out from the lateral geniculate and travel in the temporal and parietal lobes before reaching their destination in the occipital lobe. Lesions in the temporal lobe may give a homonymous superior field defect if the optic radiations are affected. Similarly, a lesion in the parietal lobe may show an inferior homonymous field defect.

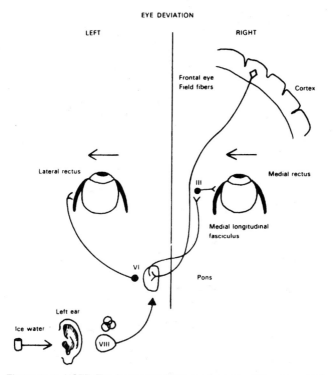

Figure 31.2. *NOTE:* The frontal eye fields exert a major influence on horizontal eye movement, each field being concerned with contralateral eye deviation. Thus, the right field causes eyes to move to the left. (The fibers cross in the pons and connect there to the extraocular muscles via the medial longitudinal fasciculus.) Both fields are constantly active, striking a balance; thus, when one is more or less active than the other, horizontal eye deviation results.

5. The *pupillary response* is affected only if fibers proximal to the lateral geniculate body or in the midbrain, the third nerve, or optic nerve fibers are damaged.
6. When one realizes the large territory needed for intact visual fields, it becomes apparent why checking visual fields is a mandatory part of every neurologic examination.

EYE DEVIATION IN NEUROLOGIC DISEASE

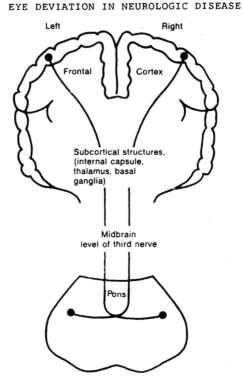

Figure 31.3. In the comatose patient with an intact brainstem, ice water in the left ear causes deviation of the eyes to the left. In the awake patient, this deviation is counteracted voluntarily, producing nystagmus to the right.

Ascending Tracts

Dorsal columns (1) carry position and vibratory sense; fibers rise ipsilaterally and cross in the medulla. These columns are laminated, but the lamination is usually of little clinical importance.

Lateral spinothalamic tract (2) carries pain and temperature sensation. These fibers cross upon entering the cord; a cord lesion affecting them produces a contralateral loss. They are laminated with sacral fibers most laterally placed. Thus, an

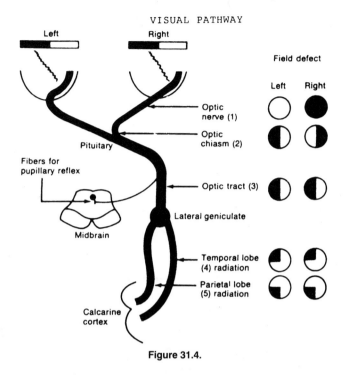

Figure 31.4.

expanding process in the center of the cord gives sacral sparing (pinprick and temperature sensory loss are least prominent in the sacral area).

Descending Tracts

Lateral corticospinal tract (3) carries motor fibers that synapse at the anterior horn cells. The fibers have already crossed in the medulla. A lesion of, or pressure upon, the corticospinal tract causes weakness, spasticity, hyperreflexia, and up-going toes.

Anterior horn cells (4) are lower motor neurons. A lesion here produces weakness, muscle wasting, fasciculations, and loss of reflexes and tone.

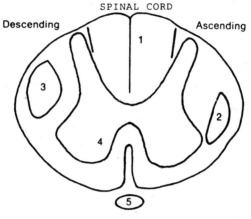

Figure 31.5.

Vascular Supply

The *anterior spinal artery* (5) supplies the entire cord except for the dorsal columns. Thus, the anterior spinal artery syndrome produces paralysis and loss of pain and temperature sense; position and vibratory sense are preserved.

Clinical Correlation

- Subacute combined system affects 1 and 3.
- Amyotrophic lateral sclerosis affects 3 and 4.
- Tabes dorsalis affects 1.
- Multiple sclerosis affect 1, 2, and 3 (alone or in combination).
- Poliomyelitis affects 4.
- Brown-Séquard syndrome (hemisection of cord) produces ipsilateral paralysis, ipsilateral loss of vibration and position sense, and contralateral loss of sensation to pinprick and temperature.

The most commonly encountered vascular syndrome affecting the medulla is the *lateral medullary (Wallenberg) syndrome* (see Chapter 6), which defines a major portion of the dysfunction that

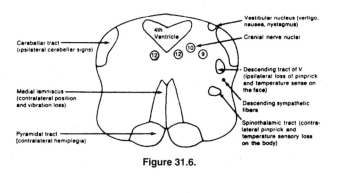

Figure 31.6.

PONS (Cranial Nerves 5 to 8)

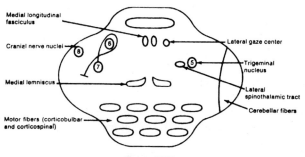

Figure 31.7.

can be seen with medullary involvement. (Medial structures are not affected: pyramids, medial lemniscus, and twelfth nerve nucleus.)

Remember that the *seventh* (facial) *nerve is not in the medulla;* thus, if facial weakness is present, there must be dysfunction at the level of the pons or above.

When *descending sympathetic fibers* are involved, an ipsilateral Horner's syndrome (ptosis, small pupil, and facial anhidrosis) results.

Cranial nerve nuclei:

- *Twelfth* (hypoglossal): Unilateral involvement of the nucleus causes fasciculations on that side; when the tongue is protruded, it deviates to the side of the lesion.

- *Tenth* (vagus) and *ninth* (glossopharyngeal): These innervate the laryngeal and pharyngeal musculature; dysphagia is prominent when they are involved.

The fibers of the seventh (facial) nerve sweep around the sixth nerve (lateral rectus) before exiting from the pons. Thus a lesion at this level often produces a VI and VII nerve paralysis on the same side.

Basic structure of the pons: Medial involvement produces motor dysfunction and internuclear ophthalmoplegia or gaze palsy to the side of the lesion. Lateral involvement causes pain and temperature dysfunction.

Vertical nystagmus is a sign of brainstem dysfunction at the level of the pontomedullary junction or upper midbrain (unless the patient is on barbiturates).

Eighth nerve nuclei include cochlear and vestibular components.

The trigeminal nerve exits from the middle of the pons and if involved at this level produces face pain and ipsilateral loss of the corneal reflex. In high pontine lesions, pain and sensory loss are contralateral to the lesion in both face and extremities. Below the high pons, pain and temperature sense are lost ipsilaterally in the face and contralaterally in the limbs.

Lesions of the *medial longitudinal fasciculus* (MLF) result in an internuclear ophthalmoplegia. If the right MLF is involved, there is difficulty with right eye adduction, as well as nystagmus in the abducting left eye when the patient looks to the left.

The most prominent disturbance in the midbrain generally involves the third nerve nucleus or exiting fibers, producing a dilated pupil and ophthalmoplegia.

Lesions affecting the area of the midbrain just below the superior colliculus produce difficulty with upward gaze, convergence, and pupillary light reflexes (Parinaud's syndrome). A tumor pressing on the superior colliculus may present in this way (e.g., pinealoma).

Lesions of the red nucleus produce contralateral ataxia and tremor (rubral tremor). The substantia nigra, located at this level, plays an important role in Parkinson's disease.

The fourth nerve nucleus is also located in the midbrain at a lower level and is seldom involved alone. When it is involved alone (e.g., due to trauma), fourth nerve injury causes a head tilt.

MIDBRAIN (Cranial Nerves 3 to 4)

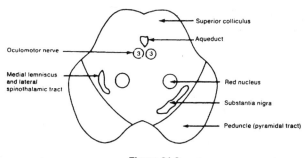

Figure 31.8.

DERMATOME SENSORY CHART

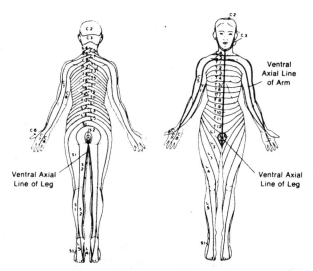

Figure 31.9. Left: Dermatomes from the posterior view. Right: The dermatomes from the anterior view. (From Keegan JJ, Garrett FD. The segmental distribution of the cutaneous nerves in the limbs of man. Anat Rec 1948;102:409. Reprinted by permission of the Wistar Institute Press, Philadelphia, Pennsylvania.)

Fibers from the optic tract concerned with the pupillary response synapse in the region of the third nerve nucleus. Lesions in the midbrain may impair pupillary reaction to direct light but leave contraction to accommodation intact.

CROSSINGS IN THE NERVOUS SYSTEM

Almost all major pathways in the nervous system cross. Much of the understanding of neuroanatomy relates to knowing where these tracts cross and thus at which level the nervous system is involved.

Suggested Reading

Gilman S, Newman S. Manter & Gatz's essentials of clinical neuroanatomy and neurophysiology. 7th ed. Philadelphia: FA Davis, 1987.

Index

Page numbers in *italics* denote figures; those followed by "t" denote tables.